About the Author

Dr. Thomas O'Connor is a board certified internist with 15 years' experience in diagnosing and treating hypogonadism in men who use anabolic steroids as well as in men who do not. He has been a pioneer in writing about and treating men who have used anabolic steroids and are suffering with side effects related to using these agents. A nearly universal side effect he sees often is anabolic steroid induced hypogonadism (ASIH), a unique form of hypogonadism unfamiliar to most other physicians. Writing as the *Anabolic Doc*, his articles have appeared in publications such as *Muscular Development, Powerlifting USA, Steroidology, and Muscle Sport Magazine;* and he is a featured author in William LLewellen's most recent *ANABOLICS, 11*[th] *Edition.* He publishes Internet videos about men's health issues regularly, often interviewing well known sports figures and other medical experts. A clinical instructor in medicine at University of Connecticut where he did his residency training, Dr. O'Connor mentors medical students interested in learning firsthand about practices like his. His reputation as a physician who takes the time to get to know his patients, viewing each one with unconditional regard, brings men to his practice from across the nation and the world. His mission now, he says, is two-fold: To promote greater awareness of medical protocols required to provide men who need it with safe and effective hormone replacement; and to warn of the burgeoning crisis of increasing AAS use across all sectors of American society. By challenging the media, professional sports and government agencies to view the latter as a public health problem, and not solely a law enforcement issue or one limited to professional athletes who cheat, he believes we may prevent the tragedy of other overlooked health crises in the past. "AAS use now is where opioids were 15 years ago," he says. It's time to take action!

isbn 978-0-9994096-0-2

AMERICA ON
Steroids

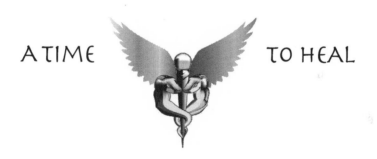

A TIME   TO HEAL

Thomas O'Connor MD

metabolic promotion LLC

mmxviii

Acknowledgements

A book doesn't write itself, nor does an author create it singlehandedly. Some very special people inspired, encouraged and supported me to bring this book to life. With gratitude, I thank:

My dear Wendy for her constant push to, "write the damn book!"; and for listening to me complain why I could not. Well, here it is, Wendy. My Mom for all she does and has done for me from the beginning. No son could be more fortunate than I, with a super-human woman for a Mom— The Anabolic Mom! Jan for his tactful fatherly guidance, and his enduring love and caring for Mom…and for the many pots of coffee. Jack, who will always be the big brother I love—the one everyone should have. And his Annie who brought her light to us all. My children Maxine and David who remind me every day that there is no greater joy than being a parent. Seeing them grow has been like watching dreams unfold.

I want to also thank Kimberly Ann DiBattista, my General Manager and office chief who masterfully administered the practice throughout this project, and who was a trusted sounding board (priceless). I will always be thankful for Kim's mom, Kimberly Ann DiBattista, who took on the task of transcribing many of the articles used in this book, even while she was ill. I am also grateful to have on my team Una McKenzie, Assistant Manager of my office; her dependability, intelligence and warmth provide a solid haven on even the craziest of days.

I wish also to acknowledge two absolutely brilliant men behind the scenes, Matt Bartone, "the Social Media Guy" and Alex Hansen, the "Master" of SEO and web workmanship. Without these guys, our word would not be heard. And finally, I want to thank Elliott Pollack, Esq. for his steadfast faith and consummate professionalism.

This book is dedicated to
Mom,
the wind beneath my wings,
and to
my patients
who keep me solidly grounded.

Table of Contents

Foreword

In many conversations with the author, Dr. Thomas O'Connor, I learned that one of many things we shared a concern about was at the same time our nation's attention is focused on perceived external threats to our country and culture, a serious internal threat is hiding in plain sight: It's hard not to notice the number of (mostly) young men who seem to achieve extraordinary muscular proportions in a short amount of time. They pack your groceries at the super market, deliver packages to your home, write you a traffic ticket, sit next to you in church and play football with your son. In unprecedented numbers, these average Joes--and some Jills--are using anabolic-androgenic steroids (AAS) and performance enhancing drugs (PEDs)—legal as well as illicit substances that offer the promise of sculpting the ideal male physique. The most widely used of these substances are anabolic steroids; therefore, all of these drugs will be referred to as AAS throughout this book, unless a reference to a specific PED was required.

AAS Business Is Booming

Because most of these drugs are illegal, using them is an underground activity. Buying them, however, is more transparent. Easily satisfied on the Internet, demand for these drugs has created an American market that is estimated to be worth $2,000,000,000 (Kellogg, 2008), with 99% of the supply coming from China (Mehaffey, 2013).

Because many data sources that measure drug abuse have not included AAS, it has been difficult to determine their prevalence .(NIDA, 2006) The National Institute of Drug Abuse estimates 2014 use at 1.3 million, while the Endocrine Society estimated the number of AAS users to be three million.

(Canavan, 2013) However, the most comprehensive study to date reports that use is actually as high as four million, with an estimated one million having become dependent on AAS. (Pope et al, 2014) These authors state, "Age-of-onset studies consistently showed that AAS use begins later than most drugs, with only 22% of users (95% confidence interval: 19–25%) starting before age 20. Applying the age-of-onset findings to national youth datasets, we estimated that among Americans currently age 13–50 years, 2.9–4.0 million have used AAS. Within this group, roughly one million may have experienced AAS dependence." A recent study reported that AAS use is a common cause of profound hypogonadism in younger men, with up to one of five men seeking treatment for this condition reporting prior AAS use. (McBride & Coward, 2016)

Studies cite use by 14% of collegiate athletes and 30% of community weight trainers, with the fastest growing group of AAS users being young men and women. The 2016 Partnership for Drug-Free Kids study found that AAS use in a group of teenagers they studied had increased from 5% to 7% compared with four previously studied periods. Nationally, they found that 1.5 million teens had tried AAS, and that half a million teens use AAS at the level of abuse each year. The Federal Drug Administration (FDA) reported similar statistics for teen use in 2016. And 11% of teens they studied reported using human growth hormone (HGH) as well—nearly double the level reported in the four preceding surveys.

Hidden Sources of AAS

Many other potentially dangerous bodybuilding products sold openly in retail stores as well as online, labeled as "dietary supplements" and promoted as either hormone products or as alternatives to AAS for increasing muscle mass and strength, actually contain AAS or steroid-like substances, synthetic hormones related to the male hormone testosterone. According to CDR Mark S. Miller, Pharm.D., a regulatory review officer at the U.S. Food and Drug Administration

(FDA), bodybuilding products that contain steroids or steroid-like substances are associated with potentially serious health risks, including liver injury. "Some of the liver injuries were life-threatening," CDR Miller says. Cara Welch, Ph.D., a senior advisor in FDA's Office of Dietary Supplement Programs, says, "Many of these products are not dietary supplements at all; they are illegally marketed, unapproved new drugs." The loophole through which these manufacturers operate legally exists only because FDA had not reviewed these products for safety, effectiveness, or quality before these companies began marketing them. (FDA, June 20, 2017)

Yes, They Are Addictive!

The drive to sculpt the perfect body at any cost explains some of the risk-taking with AAS, but it is not the full story, according to Dr. Thomas O'Connor, the author of this groundbreaking book. A record-holding powerlifter himself, and a board certified medical internist with a special interest in men's health and anabolic steroid recovery, Dr. O'Connor presents the case for intervening medically in the use of AAS and for more enlightened public policy toward use. Leaving the legal and moral proscriptions to others, he describes the many adverse health effects of using these drugs, and provides evidence that there is a point at which AAS use can no longer be seen as a free choice—namely, the point at which a user has become dependent or addicted, which occurs in 15%–30% of users. Thus, he argues, because we are witnessing a burgeoning epidemic, we must view AAS use in the same enlightened way we now view other substance abuse; that is, from a public health perspective, and not exclusively as a moral or law enforcement issue.

In this book, you will learn how the cycling protocol in which users go on and off AAS can render them so dependent on these drugs that in order to avoid the distress of withdrawal, they continue to use, sometimes adding other potentially harmful drugs, including opioids, to the mix in an attempt to counteract withdrawal effects. It is not known how many cycles it takes for users to get to the point of addiction or to experience potentially

11

irreversible harm to major organs. It is clear, however, that when a user reaches his individual tipping point, he can become trapped in AAS cycling from which he cannot exit, however much he may want to.

The Call to Action

An additional concern is that users are being exploited not only by illicit suppliers of AAS of increasingly uncertain quality, but also by some in the legitimate supplements industry whose products, as noted above, may also contain undisclosed AAS or, despite their high cost, may be virtually useless. This experienced physician's strongest criticism is of some in the medical profession itself—those doctors among the "anti-aging" professionals who prescribe these drugs in an unethical and potentially harmful manner. When he wrote about the foregoing concerns in his regular column in a popular muscle magazine, it was the last time Dr. O'Connor was published by that magazine.

Known to his readers as the Anabolic Doc since 2005, he has been writing about the unique health issues encountered by AAS users in publications dedicated to the strength athlete. His straight-talk articles address such topics as how organs are affected by AAS, and how psychological and social forces encourage use and addiction. Noting that, because of their distrust of doctors, users are reluctant to seek medical help for symptoms or to cease using, Dr. O'Connor encourages his fellow physicians to become more knowledgeable about AAS and clinical protocols that have been shown to alleviate symptoms and to restore users to health, as well as to support cessation. Simply telling a patient to "get off the juice" does not, in his view, meet the standard for either ethical or evidence- based support for cessation of AAS. The anonymized case studies you will read illustrate how the alternative—non-judgmental, evidence-based treatment protocols—made it possible for many patients to counteract harms caused by their AAS use, and to safely and successfully cease using. By similarly encouraging users to come out of the shadows and seek medical treatment, Dr. O'Connor believes that physicians can perform a significant role in prevention; they can provide a safe and effective alternative to the mythic underground "bro-science" —the risky brew of online and locker room advice on which users rely, and which facilitates continuing use, often at dangerous levels.

Because decades of flashy headlines about cheating athletes, legal and professional sanctions, classroom lectures, congressional hearings and generic drug rehab programs have failed to stem the growth of AAS use, this book is also a call to action by the media, professional sports, politicians, and government organizations, all of whom the author describes as either underperforming or missing in action: "Addressing the profound present and future effects of AAS use and curtailing its growth demands a contribution from *each* of these stakeholders—action beyond their own self interest."

The depth and breadth of information in this unprecedented book should be sufficient to motivate each of them to take action now.

Kathleen Hoekstra PhD LCSW

References

Canavan, N. Endocrine society pumped up to raise steroid abuse awareness, *Medscape*, Dec. 17, 2013

DEA. What is the scope of steroid use in the United States? US Drug Enforcement Administration, NIDA. Anabolic steroid abuse. https://www.drugabuse.gov/pubications/research-reports/anabolic-steroid-abuse. Aug. 1, 2006

DEA. Caution: Bodybuilding products can be risky, US Dept of Health and Human Services, website, June 20, 2017.

Kellogg, S. Juiced: congress, steroids, and the law, *Washington Lawyer*, May 2008

McBride, J.A., Coward, R. Recovery of spermatogenesis following testosterone replacement therapy or anabolic-androgenic steroid use. *Asian J Androl*. 2016 May-June; 18(3): 373–380. Published online 2016 Feb 23. doi: 10.4103/1008-682X.173938 PMCID:

Mehaffey, J. Criminals control a large part of world sports says Mehaffey, *Reuters,* Mar. 16, 2011.

Partnership for Drug-Free Kids. Taylor Hooton Foundation, 2016

Pope, HG et al. The lifetime prevalence of anabolic-androgenic steroid use and dependence in Americans: current best estimates, *Am J Addict,* 2014;23:371–377

1

Why I Wrote This Book

Disclaimer: The purpose of this book is to educate and is in no way intended to be a substitute for professional medical advice. All cases have been anonymized so that no particular patient is identifiable.

It's Not So Lonely at the Top

The reality of the sports world is that the bar has now been raised so high that, despite drug testing regulations, many athletes will use PEDs—primarily AAS—in order to improve their performance. Harrison "Skip" Pope, professor of psychiatry at Harvard's Mc- Lean Hospital, an avid weightlifter himself and an acknowledged expert on AAS, refers to keeping drugs out of sports as a "Sisyphean task." He states, "Those of us who do research in this area are all quite cynical about the magnitude of doping in sports and feel that it is all probably much greater than is generally believed by the public," he says. "It's also extremely difficult to control, and even with the best control, it still persists". (Butterworth, 2017 In 2014, *Pharmacy Times* reported that six out of 10 Olympic athletes used PEDs. (Wick, 2014) For a recent testing period, the World

Anti-Drugging Association (WADA reported that 600 doping violations were found in Olympic athletes they tested. (Berkowitz and Meko, 2016 In contrast to WADA, which maintains testing samples for 8 years, professional sports in the United States avoid such extensive anti-doping programs as players' unions and collective bargaining agreements prevent extensive testing. (Wick, 2014)

So, despite official denials, AAS use by professional and Olympic athletes is a significant part of the overall AAS picture. However, it's clear now that these athletes do not represent the majority of AAS users. Most of the men I treat, and for whom I write, are regular guys—and some women—who just love to look and feel great. The vast majority are not involved in athletics. However, they do share in the pro's exposure to the many serious health effects of these drugs. What they do NOT share, in all likelihood, is the support of knowledgeable physicians who can warn them about and counter some of these.

In this book, I will be addressing current and potential AAS users, and those who love them; health professionals and policy makers—many of whom need or want to understand more about these dangerous drugs and the people who use them. I will attempt to make the case that better understanding of AAS will not only help *all* users to protect their own health, but will also arm physicians to support them in this. A related goal is to encourage more rational public policy regarding AAS. That is, recognizing and responding to AAS use as a burgeoning public health epidemic and not exclusively a law enforcement issue—as an epidemic which is already threatening the health of millions of Americans, including a growing number of teens (Partnership for Drug-Free Kids, 2016). I hope each of the reader-stakeholders I appeal to in this book will recognize the role they can play to combat it.

The chapters in this book represent my writing as the *Anabolic Doc* in *Muscular Development, Powerlifting USA, Muscle Sport Magazine, Steroidology* and *Powerlifting Watch,* as well as in Bill Llewellen's classic book, *Anabolics.* In those articles, I wrote to alert users to the health effects of anabolic steroids, and to inform them about safe and effective medically supervised protocols to address these and to support medically supervised withdrawal and cessation. Now, as then, I remind my readers that I am writing to educate, to inform, and not to treat. One must always be mindful that medical treatment should be unique to each individual, and should never take place without thorough assessment and accurate diagnosis of a problem, and discussion of all possible solutions between a patient and their physician.

Where Do AAS Come From?

As much as 99% of all AAS are made in China, where AAS are not illegal. (Mehaffey, 2013) The US is now the largest outlet in the world for AAS, as well as many other banned or counterfeit drugs. And, because China has enjoyed US Most Favored Nation status since 2000, these products may also enter the US either tax free or with a very low tariff, often mislabeled as innocuous dietary ingredients or concealed in the bottom of large drums of legal supplements. Because drug dogs can't detect steroids like they can narcotics, a package suspected to contain steroids would have to be tested in a lab. The delay gives smugglers time to destroy documents or simply move their operation. No major illegal AAS importer has yet to serve jail time; however, one has been deported back to China and has promised to "never again import or export AAS to America". (US DOJ, June 2015)

Who Is Using AAS?

Over the past 15 years or so, researchers and media outlets have occasionally attempted to tell the broader story of increasing steroid use by the average man or woman, including police and armed services personnel. (Bernton, 2010) However, these intermittent reports have been eclipsed by long-running front page stories of multimillion dollar athletes who cheat to win. At the same time when politicians jostle to get before the cameras to shame these offenders in this modern morality play, Harvard University professors who publish articles and give interviews about the far wider prevalence and dangers of these drugs fail

17

to gain much traction either within the medical profession or from anyone in public or government service. And Chinese steroids continue to flood the US, as increasing numbers of young men—and women— seek the perfect body.

Most beginning users who get younger every year are naive or dismissive of the dangers of AAS. Captive as youth ever was to fantasies of immortality, the majority of high school students persistently believe that steroids are not dangerous or addictive. (PDFK, 2016) Still, despite the fact that the government's own official figures on AAS use clearly indicate that a significant number of people—including school aged youths—are taking dangerous risks with their health, the bulk of government funding continues to be spent on law enforcement rather than on treatment and prevention. (Blumenson & Nilson, 1998)

In a 2013 interview, Dr. Shalender Bhasin of Harvard University described the majority of AAS users as cosmetically motivated average men and women risking their health for the sake of a buff image. To address the "tsunami" of serious AAS health effects gathering in our corner gyms, he called for physicians to become more knowledgeable about these drugs and about how to support safe and effective cessation. (Canavan, 2013) Certainly, Dr. Bhasin's pull-no- punches statements were a strong call to arms for the medical profession. Similar articles, which I will discuss in subsequent chapters, have appeared in other prominent medical journals before and since then to encourage physicians to take a stronger role. In February 2017, *Time Magazine* published a well documented article quoting other distinguished AAS experts who also warned about the prevalence and dangers of steroids use. *It is important to note that all of the above sources converge on the view that AAS use is more widespread and potentially dangerous than is popularly perceived.*

So, every now and then, if you know where to look, you can find professional and popular media reports indicating the dangers and prevalence of AAS use. But, to date, there is nothing near the coverage one would expect regarding a burgeoning public health epidemic. After I stop shaking my head at this, I begin to wonder: Why would such serious, repeated, reliable warnings continue to be ignored?

When we heard about Zika virus, the nation went on high alert, with the media as well as the government playing an important role in disseminating needed information to keep people safe. The result was pressure on Congress to appropriate timely emergency funding to stem the epidemic. Which it did. Similarly, because the opioids/heroin epidemic has received more than passing media coverage, we have greater understanding of the elements that created the epidemic, and some insights into addressing it. So, while solutions will not be immediate, some crucial points of intervention have been identified. This experience has demonstrated how critical widespread dissemination of information is for crisis intervention, how such heightened focus can provide useful information to policy makers and professionals as well as to the public. On the other hand, the fact that the opioids epidemic had been well underway —claiming and ruining many lives years before it received this critical level of attention—is an example of the price we pay for delay, for less than timely recognition of a burgeoning epidemic.

The Elephant in the Locker Room

I think a number of factors have contributed to the less than adequate current response to the AAS threat to public health. One element is the narrow media focus on doping in professional sports, which has contributed to most people believing that AAS are used only by cheating athletes. So, many folks are still asleep, waiting to be woke. Another reason is that people who use AAS shun the spotlight because they fear legal and employment consequences, as well as the potential loss of their AAS supplies. As a result, even when users do encounter medical problems related to AAS, or when they want to stop using, they avoid seeing doctors—and are not always honest when they do see them. And, in all fairness, not all doctors signal that they are open to hearing about AAS- related problems, despite the fact that safe, effective clinical protocols for addressing

19

AAS-related health issues and for helping users cease using are available. In subsequent chapters, I will discuss these protocols, which are recommended by major medical organizations like the Endocrine Society, the Cleveland Clinic, and Harvard University School of Medicine.

Yes, there is some evidence of private and government support for drug education programs in schools. However, the increase in teen AAS use indicates that this has not had the intended impact. Where AAS drug testing of students—a strongly contested civil rights issue— has been tried, it has often been an admitted failure. In 2015, the state of Texas unfunded a school testing program which, although it cost the taxpayer $10 million dollars over 8 years, yielded only 40 positives in that time. Several other states have reported similarly low yields. It's simply too costly to do legally questionable widespread testing, and too easy for kids to beat the system. (Cook, 2015)

Where is the sports industry in the hidden-in-plain-sight AAS epidemic? Major League Baseball (MLB) is a major funder of Partnership for Drug-Free Kids, whose activities are primarily focused on educational programs—a laudable contribution by MLB. Still, it seems disproportionate to the wealth they have accrued—occasionally pillorying a few errant players while, as numerous observers believe, many other players are using PEDs.

Similarly, many who are familiar with professional sports are cynical about the NFL's intention to fully honor their 2013 agreement to test players. (Selig and Gupta, 2017) It's reasonable to suspect that it is in US Olympics' and professional sports' corporate interests to define the AAS problem as poor choices by a few of their athletes and some high school athletes—and not as the pervasive public health problem it actually is.

And the media? What role could they be playing to promote timely response this burgeoning epidemic? The media loves a good story. They need a steady stream of these to survive. But, with the ongoing decline in the ranks of investigative journalists as media budgets continue to shrink, don't expect the media to lead the charge. It is, unfortunately, too often in their interest to follow the most popular elephant into the room. As noted earlier, an article about the prevalence and dangers of steroids pops up here and there, but nothing in from Bob Woodward or Michael Moore as yet.

And How About Our Politicians?

As a former bodybuilder himself, I would have thought that Arnold "the Gov" Schwarzenegger might have weighed in. But then I recalled his annual cult event, The Arnold Expo. The roar of the crowd… Farther up the political food chain, the response is no more encouraging: millions of taxpayer dollars spent on the prolonged Barry Bonds case has demonstrated the government's selective appetite for addressing steroids use. At the same time when scant government resources were targeted for research or treatment of AAS use by four million Americans, the Department of Justice spared no expense in their effort to convict Bonds of perjury and obstruction of justice for his testimony to a Grand Jury (ironically, the first time anyone was charged with perjury for providing a truthful answer). And my local legislators? I've written to them. Nice responses. So, the AAS epidemic has many facets, many faces, and many missed opportunities.

References

Berkowitz, B and Meko, T. Stronger, faster, longer and higher… a look at the summer Olympics, *Washington Post*, June 28, 2016

Bernton, H & Meko, T. Stronger, faster, longer and higher... *Washington Post*, June 28, 2016

Blumenson, E and Nilson E. The drug wars hidden economic agenda, *The Nation*, Mar. 9, 1998

Butterworth, T. Steroids are more dangerous than you think, *Newsweek*, June 2017

Cook, B. Why testing HS students (for steroids) is a big fat failure, *Forbes*, June 2015

Heid, M. Why men have more body image issues than ever, *Time Magazine*, Jan. 5, 2007

Partnership for Drug-Free Kids. *Taylor Hooton Foundation*, 2016

Selig, R, Gupta S. What the NFL could learn about drug testing from the UFC, *CNN* Feb. 6, 2017

US Department of Justice. Chinese national pleads guilty to conspiracy, *FDA Release* Dec. 4, 2015

Wick, J. PEDs: a new reality in sports? *Pharm Times* Mar 2014

2

The Luckiest
Doc in the World

It was not long ago that I submitted my first article as the   Anabolic Doc—"Big Medicine". In it, I reflected on one of those days when I again deeply considered what I do, where I've come. It was a day of poignant memory and gratitude as I was presented with two gifts. The first gift was another lifter patient who makes the trek from the Midwest to see me; and the other gift, from an old friend, was a picture of me back in the day, circa 1984, when I was 20 years old and about 230+ pounds—a poster boy for the Adonis complex.

I remember exactly what I was thinking when that picture was taken: I was only concerned about being big...and lifting BIG, back then, up at the Old School "townie" gyms I trained at outside Syracuse University. Sometimes, I felt like an impostor student on "The Hill" because all I really wanted to do was to get to the gym and squat more—or at least weigh more—on days like the one on which that picture was taken by Dave, who has since remained one of my dearest friends. Forget the nights waking up to eat half sticks of butter, not to lose weight! I wanted to be a "lifter," and I would do almost anything to be accepted and respected by those I trained with. Those were the days when I spent a hell of a lot more of my day in the gym than the library. Over the years, those motivations and that behavior have changed. But some of the feelings still return when I meet a new lifter patient.

Today, as I was preparing to examine a new patient (just like me, back in the day, although much larger, stronger, and better looking), while I was wheeling out my ECG machine to check his heart, I had to stop in the hall for a moment and take a deep breath. I smiled and shook my head with self-approval as I recognized that, as far as I'd come from those halcyon days, now working in an honored profession I truly love and have been well trained for, I still have the same passion for this sport and the same respect for the people who practice it. Many of my patients remind me of the men I used to train heavy with back in the day. So, while we talk easily about lifting and share our stories, I also get to practice my other passion, medicine, with the brothers and sisters of iron. Anything I can do for them feels like giving back to those who shared so generously with me. I can imagine that the scenario I'm painting might prompt the reader to think, "steroids?" Beyond inquiring about use for diagnostic purposes, or cautioning patients who use these agents or are considering using them, there is no place for such discussion in my professional role. I don't judge, I heal.

FOTOS: The Doc with Joe Ladnier in video on Heart Health; Doc's "Know Your Labs" video; with Prof. Fred Hatfield (Dr. Squat) talking in video about powerlifting "back in the day".

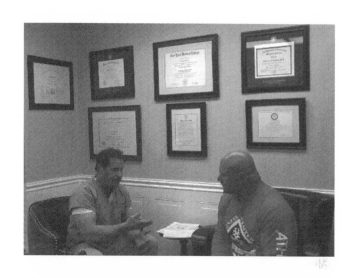

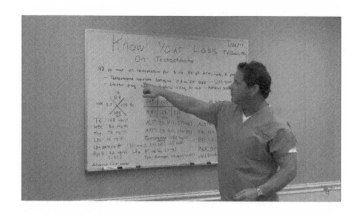

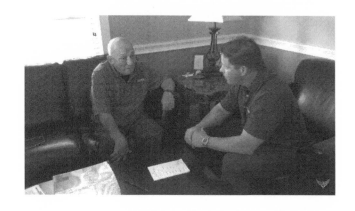

3

Steroids on Synthol

On my last trip to the Arnold bodybuilding expo in 2012, I thought I saw it all: tons of guys on gear and feats of unimaginable strength on stage, in the side rooms, and at the Animal Cage. But this year blew all the things I saw in the past away. I witnessed a man rep-out with 600 pounds raw on the bench— easy! The guys are bigger, faster, and stronger; and more women than ever appear to be geared up. At my Metabolic Doc booth, I heard stories from dozens of men who have been using AAS and who are now concerned about their health. This is why I attend the Arnold, so such dialogue is par for the course, but this year something new was added to the conversations: I had at least 10 men tell me that they are now using synthol and other muscle site enhancement oils (SEOs) in addition to steroids. I knew that SEOs were out there, but I thought they were limited to professional bodybuilders who used them in a limited fashion. Was I in for a rude awakening! On my plane ride home, I knew I needed to research SEOs for an article for *Muscle Sport Magazine*. Except for case reports of horror stories about self-injected synthol and other oils, there is little solid evidence-based medical literature regarding SEOs. I have based this chapter on a few of the articles I was able to locate (they are listed here and at the end of this chapter)

(Ghandourah, S et al, 2012; Ludlow, N, 2015).

The most commonly used SEO is synthol, which was developed in the mid-1990s by a German bodybuilder. Synthol is a blend of 85% oil (medium-chain triglycerides), 7.5% lidocaine (local anesthetic), and 7.5% benzyl alcohol (sterilizer). We have all seen those incredible photos from Brazil, of men on synthol but until recently, the use of synthol had not been seen often in the average American gym. Taking synthol is a quick and easy way to look big and muscular without actually having to lift weights or become strong by training hard. Hence, its appeal is to bodybuilders who don't want to do the really heavy lifting. Curiously, in Latin American countries, men who use synthol and develop all manner of what we might think of as freakish looks are not always seen in that way. Perhaps use is so widespread that the imitation factor is at work; maybe even the outdo factor.

The way in which synthol is used also suggests in some a form of body dysmorphia. However, my primary job as a physician, and not a psychiatrist, is not to assess or judge motivations but to bring attention to the medical consequences of using these agents. And SEOs like synthol can certainly lead to some very dangerous consequences. Nick Ludlow, a respected fitness guru, has provided what I think is a thorough and accurate description of the potential side effects related to SEOs. Here is his list, along with some of my own edits:

- Deformed and unnaturally shaped muscles
- Purpuras, which occur when small blood vessels leak blood under the skin
- Nerve damage
- Infection, which is very common and can lead to serious chronic local infections requiring in-hospital intravenous antibiotics and multiple surgeries
- Localized redness, swelling, pressure, and pain in and around the injected muscle group(s)
- Abcesses, which are collections of pus in any part of the body that, in most cases, cause swelling and inflammation

- Skin ruptures
- Complete halt to natural muscle regeneration
- Induration/sclerosis, which are hardened patches of tissue in the skin or mucous membranes
- Cysts, which are closed pockets or pouches of tissue filled with air, fluid, pus, or other material (these may be named according to the injected material—for example, paraffinoma as a result of injecting paraffin
- Cystic scar tissue
- Pulmonary artery occlusion/pulmonary embolism, which is the blockage or closing of the artery that carries blood from the heart to the lungs (THIS CAN BE DEADLY!)
- Vacuolation, which is the formation of small cavities in cellular tissue and which creates a "Swiss cheese" pattern within the muscle
- Vasculitis, the inflammation of blood vessels
- Sclerosing lipogranulomatosis, which is a subcutaneous inflammatory and fibrosing reaction that occurs with regional lymphadenopathy (that is, irregular lymph nodes)
- Fibrosis, or the thickening, stiffening, and scarring of connective tissue
- Hard edema, which is a hardening of fluid build-up in body tissue
- Lymphangitis, or infection of the lymph vessels throughout the body, which is typically caused by complications from bacterial infections
- Fistulas, which are abnormal connections between an organ, vessel, or intestine and another structure
- Cerebral stroke, in which blood flow (oxygen and

nutrients) to all or part of the brain ceases

- Myocardial infarction/heart attack, in which blood flow (oxygen and nutrients) to all or part of the heart ceases (Ludlow, 2015)

In addition to this list, Nick has provided a useful bibliography of synthol case reports. We have all seen the grotesque photos of synthol users and read the horror stories. These make it hard to believe that so many people are now adding synthol to steroids. Is it really happening? Are steroids now on synthol? Is this the future? What's next?! I'm still trying to get my head around it. I wonder if social media may be playing a role here: Could the guys who, only a few years ago, wanted to have a sexy photo or a cool "super-human" avatar for their Facebook page now want to look like an actual super human in person? Enter steroids on synthol. To achieve anything close to such an appearance using only steroids, you must not only take them but also train hard, eat right, and tolerate the side effects. Whereas with SEOs, it appears that guys think they can get that perfect body despite poor genes or less training, and even with less steroids.

Whatever the reason, there is no question that AAS and synthol each have their dangers, so please do your research. A direct conversation with your physician will tell you whether he or she is knowledgeable about AAS. Staying in the shadows with your AAS use could cost you your health— or even your life.

References

Ghandourah, S, Hofer, MJ, Kießling, A, El-Zayat, B, Schofer, MB. Painful muscle fibrosis following synthol injections in a bodybuilder: a case report, *Journal of Medical Case Reports,* 2012 Aug 20;6:248.

Ludlow, N. Dangers of synthol oil injections for muscle enhancement, TigerFitness.com, June 2015

4

Time to Be
Responsible

Dear Lifter,

We have all read conflicting articles on what to do and not to do during a cycle to help improve your results. But there are few articles that identify very serious side effects from a medical perspective. That's where I come in. As a physician, my job is not to judge the choices people make but rather to identify how some of the choices they make can contribute to serious medical conditions. I'm not just talking about beginning users, but also the veterans in the sport. I have said from the beginning of my stint as the Anabolic Doc that if you take the AAS path, you have to be fully aware of the consequences and you should do all that you can to prevent health problems down the road—not only to protect yourself but also for the welfare of your partner, your spouse, and your family who are dependent on you.

Time to Be Responsible

It is imperative to understand that if you are a strength athlete who has decided to go to the dark side and incorporate AAS into your program, I expect you to be responsible for taking care of your own health. I'm not talking about today or tomorrow, but about the next 20-plus years of your life. The problem with many strength athletes is that they do not think about long-term consequences. They only think of what is happening right now, today. But remember: You reap what you sow. The decision you make today may come and bite you on the ass like a rabid pit bull tomorrow. I expect you to do your part to take responsibility for your health.

Not Getting Blood Work Done

This item is the most important piece of information that I am going to give you. No matter who your doctor is, blood work should be done at least twice per year. This includes a full panel of tests, including your cholesterol, both high-density lipoprotein (HDL) and low-density lipoprotein (LDL). Your blood pressure, triglycerides, liver values, and kidney function should also be monitored regularly, along with any other factors present in your family and personal health history. This is the bare minimum needed to know how your organs are functioning. How do you know what is going on with your body if you don't get checked at least a couple times per year? Some bodybuilders are very responsible about this, but not enough of them are: It's my guess that no more than 20% of those who use steroids are this responsible. The biggest offenders in this area are powerlifters who have been put off by bad experiences with physicians in the past. For you, I have three words: Get over it! Find a doctor who has read the research, has an open mind, and is clear that his or her job is to heal…not judge. In my office, I have seen world-class powerlifters who have been using steroids for close to 15 years and yet have never gotten their blood work done! In my opinion, that's the single most irresponsible thing you could do.

You can't do something like go on 30 cycles over a decade and then think, "Hey maybe I should get some blood work done to see if my liver isn't bloated like a dead horse's." If this is your current mental state, you are going to pay the piper and pay him handsomely if you don't step up and take care of your health. *When reality hits you in the face, you will wish you listened to the Anabolic Doc and the message he tried to convey!* I truly care for your health and want you to be the best competitive athlete you can be. At the same time, I want you to realize that if you are taking prescription-strength drugs to reach those goals, that 50 mg of Thai Dbol pills you chugged down this morning with your oatmeal was not a handful of Red Hots (I loved that candy when I was a kid!) but a serious medication. Some are more serious than others; you will see this when we discuss insulin and thyroid drugs later in the book.

You may think you are badass because you weigh 200 pounds with 8% body fat, but listen to me closely for a minute. When one of your organs fails, or another major ailment takes you down, you will see pretty quickly that you are not made of steel. The biggest badass can be brought to his knees when organ failure prevents his body from functioning the way it should. So, please, don't let your stats make you think you are indestructible—even if you can bench press 600 pounds or if your arms are 23 inches now.

Using Underground Steroids: Consider the Source

I can see some expert lifters reading this now and saying, "This guy doesn't know the reality of the scene, man—this doc is out of his environment." I've have been in the powerlifting trenches longer than most of you have been alive. I saw the anabolic pharmacology underground scene in the old-school gyms when your mother was still tying your shoelaces. And I have seen it go from bad to worse as the supply chain shifted with Operation Gear Grinder back in 2005. (USA Today, 2008) The Feds put a halt to much of the veterinary-grade gear coming out of Mexico that supplied 90% of the black market in this country— Quality Vet, Denkall, Animal Power, Brovel, Tornel, SYD Group, and others who were the major players in the US steroid black market. An unintended consequence of this halt was that it ultimately spawned a massive increase in clandestine labs and new import sources from even more uncertain sources and countries. The result? *Buyers have no idea where their gear is coming from or*

33

what it contains. You could have some guy making this stuff in his garage, in an environment that resembles a slum in Calcutta. This is what you want to inject into your body? No wonder so many guys are getting abscesses like it's in style. Cleanliness is of utmost importance not only so you don't get an abscess that erupts like Mount Vesuvius but also for your organ health. If you think you are doing your kidneys any favors by injecting dirty gear, think again, my friend.

Didn't you ever wonder what years of injecting dirty shit could do to your organs? The lack of sterility is only one of the problems you could run into. What about metals, carcinogens, and contaminants? We all know that virtually all of the raw powders that these underground labs use come in illegally from China. If you've watched the news over the last few years, you know that all Chinese manufacturing doesn't have the best reputation. The lead paint used in children's toys? The melamine in the baby formulas? Close to 300,000 Chinese babies becoming ill because of this? Many of those babies died, and several hundred remained in critical condition because of major kidney shutdown . (Buckley, 2008) If these Chinese entrepreneurs were willing to cut corners to save money risking a major health crisis like this in their own country, how would you rate Chinese steroids and supplements manufacturers' compassion toward bodybuilders living in the US? The correct answer is LOW!

Consider also the case of polychlorinated biphenyls (PCBs, which are compounds developed in 1929 for a wide range of industrial uses, and which consist of close to 210 different chemicals. The problem with this stuff is that it is super resilient; it takes forever to break down. (Mayes et al, 1998) This is where it gets juicy. The International Agency for Research on Cancer has stated several times that exposure to PCBs can increase your chances of developing cancer— listen up here, folks—specifically, liver and kidney cancer. If this doesn't make you sit up and take notice, I don't know what will. A number of studies have shown that many underground AAS labs brew products that contain an abundance of heavy metals and other contaminants. To really make your hair stand on end, read any of the research on this by noted AAS expert, Bill Llewellyn.

A study worth reading, published in the *British Medical Journal,* found that "the potential for serious adverse health consequences due to poor manufacturing of products is not generally perceived as a major issue" among AAS users. (Kimergård and McVeigh, 2014) Think about that for a minute more, my friends: not only do you not know the conditions in which your underground gear is made, you also don't even know the country from which the powder is coming. Maybe the same company that is pumping hormone powders onto the black market is making a carcinogenic chemical in the same manufacturing equipment. I bet you didn't think of that scenario the last time you bought a bottle of underground Deca from your boy "Big Jimmy" in the change room at your local gym.

You're going to tell me that it's hard to get real pharmaceutical gear. That American-made products that were available in the 80s and 90s, and all the goodies from Europe, are no longer a viable option. I understand that those in the US who choose to use steroids see themselves as being between a rock and a hard place. That doesn't change the fact that you could be introducing potent carcinogens into your system via injection because a corrupt supplier in Shanghai doesn't care if your raw hormone powder contains impurities that will give you cancer in 10 years.

References

Buckley, C. More than 54,000 affected by milk scandal, *Reuters,* September 2008.

DEA leads largest steroid bust in history, *USA Today*, September 24, 2007

Kimergård, A, McVeigh, J. Environments, risk and health harms; a qualitative investigation..., *BMJ Open*, 2014 Jun. 4;(4):e005275

Llewellyn, W. Counterfeit analysis report, *Muscular Development,* September 3, 2009. http://www.musculardevelopment .com/articles/chemical-enhancement/1739-counterfeit

35

-analysis-report.html

Mayes, BA et al. Comparative carcinogenicity in Sprague-Dawley rats of the polychlorinated biphenyl mixtures, *Toxicol Sci,* 1998 Jan;42(1):62-76.

5

Anabolic Sisters

This chapter is dedicated to JS, a very special fan of the Anabolic Doc. It was her email that was the impetus for this chapter. JS, I hope that you enjoy my response.

I was vacationing on the beaches of Maine this summer when JS's e-mail came in. It was one e-mail of many I received that week from women around the world asking me to talk about the issues faced by women in bodybuilding and strength training. Some were pretty aggressive about feeling left out of my discussions, but JS was both polite and assertive—and that's why she gets the shout-out today. It's no secret that I focus on the Big Boys of the iron game, so it's about time that I open up the Anabolic Doc's waiting room to the sisters who train just as hard.

Of course, not all women lifters are using AAS but, when they do, the effects are similar to those seen in men in terms of muscle tissue hypertrophy and adipose tissue atrophy: women also get stronger and leaner by adding AAS to their training regimen. There are some gender differences in the medical consequences of these drugs, but in the sense that they can be serious, irreversible, and even deadly, downstream these consequences are generally equal.

Just as is the case for men, there are many different reasons why women choose to use AAS, from simply wanting to improve their looks to wanting an extra edge in athletics and onstage. There is also a medical condition that can contribute to both men and women using steroids— body dysmorphia, a variant of obsessive-compulsive disorder that bears similarities to an eating disorder. One study found that many women bodybuilders suffer from both body dysmorphia and an eating disorder (see chapter 8 on body dysmorphia). Other research has found that many women use steroids because they feel a need to protect themselves (for example, victims of rape). Such reports are found in studies of women weightlifters, where twice as many of those who had been raped acknowledged using AAS and/or other purported muscle-building drugs compared to those who had not been raped. Moreover, almost all of those who had been raped reported a marked increase in their bodybuilding activities after the attack. Their bodybuilding activity was supported by their belief that being bigger and stronger would discourage further attacks by making themselves seem more intimidating. (Goldfield, 2009; Hansen et al, 2017)

In another study involving 75 women, 10 reported being raped as their reason for using AAS to increase muscle strength and size. The rape victims in most cases believed they would never be able to trust a man again and replaced these relationships with bodybuilding activities. Of the 10 rape victims, five said that prior to the attack they had no intention of ever using AAS and believed these were a sign of weakness and unwillingness to achieve goals through hard work. (Gruber and Pope, 2000) The steroid-using women I have seen in the clinic have presented with all the classic side effects of AAS, and they were very open about which drugs they use. Notable is the fact that women who are interested in competing tend to use real testosterone because they try to limit the androgenic effects of AAS.

The list of these known androgenic effects of AAS specific to women includes:

- Hair loss and facial hair growth
- Facial structural changes with nose and brow growth
- Loss of breasts
- Voice changes toward a man's octave
- Clitoral enlargement (proportional to strength of gear)

In addition to these side effects, the women I treat tend to have more severe abnormalities in liver function, immunity and lipid changes, and hypertension than those found in men using the same drugs. These observations suggest that perhaps the internal chemistry of a woman is more averse to making hormones. I have not seen any woman in my practice experience a heart attack—as I have with my male patients—but I am sure that if a woman takes AAS long enough, her cardiovascular risks will approach those of men who use. Coronary artery plaque buildup will progress in any person. So, just as is the case with their brothers in iron, there is no free lunch for these women. They should understand the risks associated with their desire to have a strong, beautiful body. One final note to my own medical colleagues: I hope that we will soon see more gender-specific research on AAS and not repeat mistakes from the past; for example, when findings in studies of men and cardiovascular disease were mindlessly projected onto women.

References

Goldfield, G. Body image, disordered eating and anabolic steroid use in female bodybuilders, *Eating Disorders,* 2009;17(3):200-210

Gruber, A.,Pope, HG. Psychiatric and medical effects of

anabolic-androgenic steroid use in women, *Psychother Psychosom,2000;69:(1)19-26*

Hanson, G et al. *Drugs and society*, 13th ed., Burlington, MA Jones & Bartlett, 2017

6

Check Out
Your
Neighborhood
Anti-Aging
Doc

No, really, check them out…carefully.

For those of you out there who did not know that you can get hooked up with AAS directly from a doctor in the US, guess what? You can buy gear like you're ordering from a Chinese menu—"I'll take a 10cc bottle of Deca, a 20cc bottle of testosterone cypionate, some Anavar pills, and can you please add some Winstrol?" And all it will cost you, above the menu price, is about 20 years of your life. They'll even throw in the likely eventual heart failure and potential kidney transplant for free. And all of this from some of your local "anti-aging" doctors. I have a steady pipeline of patients coming to see me from these docs. Some of these docs from whom I am getting these "referrals" are getting ready to do some aging in jail. Yes, I have formed an opinion on medical "anti-aging" establishments.

Circa 2005, we opened up the first-ever concierge/retainer medical practice in central Connecticut. To build the practice, I thought I'd take a look at anti-aging and medicine. I don't know how I missed the buzz in residency at a university hospital program as good as UConn. Might have been the 30+-hour shifts and the bleeding from the eyes in this Level 1 Medical Center as I was trying to help patients actually make it to their old age. Anyway, I had some catching up to do, so off I went for a weekend trip to Vegas to catch the next wave—anti-aging medicine— at a major international seminar. Sitting in on some of the human growth hormone (HGH) lectures and finally hearing enough bullshit that contradicted basic medical science—and seeing no real evidence for any of their regimens—I decided to salvage the trip, hit Vegas hard for the remaining part of that day and night, and leave a couple of days early. Too bad it's not true that what happens in Vegas stays in Vegas. The BS that happened there certainly didn't stay there but seems to have been carried home on Sunday night by many of the starry-eyed docs I left behind me. The only difference between much of what's now called "anti-aging" medicine and snake oil is that snake oil is less dangerous. And cheaper.

Early in my practice, the damage from AAS I saw was caused by the patients themselves, with their use of underground/illicit gear. Later, I had an influx of equally sick men, toxic from medical anti-aging treatment. I still can't believe that there are doctors in this country that will prescribe 500 mg a week of testosterone cypionate, Anavar, and Deca—all together, and for years. I have even treated a 68-year-old man who was on this regimen from an anti-aging clinic. Again, it's one thing that this type of AAS use occurs in the street, but by the hand of a real doctor? I know that not all of the anti-aging doctors practice this way, but here's the thing: It appears that it is ONLY anti-aging docs that are doing this. Even the title "anti-aging" rubs me the wrong way. Is anyone really looking to "anti-age" with HGH, thyroid hormones, steroids, or even scarier things such as telomerase inhibitors—and for $20,000 per year?

7

No Free Lunch

After years of writing as the Anabolic Doc and providing medical care for lifters, seeing the number of men (and a few women) lifter patients who have joined my practice indicated that there are substantial numbers who want to maintain their health while pursuing their passion. Letting it be known that I welcomed strength athletes seems to have been the medical example of "If you build it, they will come." In addition to these healthy strength athletes, a significant number of patients are coming to see me from the so-called anti-aging clinics. It's scary to see what some of these "medical" establishments do (and don't do) for their patients—customers, really. The federal government has been closing down many of the "anti-aging/rejuvenation" clinics all over the US. I'm hardly "pro Big Brother," but thank God some of these places are getting shut down.

Many of my anti-aging clinic rescues have actually never even spoken to a doctor, even while receiving FedEx boxes of steroids from these clinics for years. And as for the "laboratory assessment" that was supposed to be done

43

during their treatment period…don't ask. The protocol for monitoring a man on steroids or testosterone is not rocket science; the physician involved should be addressing the following basics that relate to the many critical medical issues encountered by steroids users as well as by men who require testosterone replacement, TRT (or he or she should not be practicing medicine):

- Simple polycythemia
- Differentiate true renal failure from a false-positive low estimated glomerular filtration rate (GFR)
- Abnormalities in lipid levels
- Abnormalities related to basic urine analysis
- Prostate warnings
- Any changes in key issues with key vital or clinical signs
- Symptoms indicating that something is going wrong...

I'm frustrated when I see so many anti-aging graduates coming in to me with existing and avoidable diseases—especially involving the heart and kidneys —that are attributable to using steroids but are completely avoidable. When patients who have come from anti-aging clinics have to be on testosterone replacement following removal of all the drugs they had been receiving, they soon report how much better they feel on their physiological dose of pharmaceutical-grade testosterone from CVS or Walgreens. In addition, many benefit from having their insurance pay the cost for their TRT because a medical need for it has been established; it's not just about being forever young.

To be clear, I'm not bashing all compounding pharmacies, but I suspect that the disreputable anti-aging clinics I'm talking about add to the list of their harms the fact that they are making gear just like many underground labs do, with bulk gear powder from China. Think of those risks! Maybe the average US doctor does not know how to deliver testosterone to you the way you would really like or need, but most sincerely have your health in mind. I see this in the calls I get from physicians who are seeking advice when they have a patient on testosterone or with a history of anabolic steroid use.

Just the other morning, I was in one of those pre-waking states, thinking about this book, when the phrase, "no free lunch" came to me. I even thought it might make a good title. (My editor talked me out of it later that day.) What I was thinking was this: Have you ever had any real achievement that came easy? No? Nor have I. I think most of us recognize that when it comes to career or relationship issues, nothing worthwhile is achieved without significant cost. But, sad to say, this fact of life is missing in the calculus of too many men, women, and teens when they are seeking their ideal body and paradoxically destroying it at the same time with AAS and other dangerous chemicals.

I spend my days talking to patients about how to achieve optimal health and training goals. It would be easy (but I would be out of a job) if we could all just juice-up and train like beasts, with no worry for our health. However, there is a big difference between achieving strength in a healthy body versus pursuing strength in ways that harm that body, and between fostering sustainable strength that enhances health, and prostituting one's health for the sake of appearing strong. I am saddened when the latter person comes to me with not only serious health problems but also regret for what they have done. I do understand that the iron world is one of extremes and sacrifice, but the sacrifice shouldn't include health. For those patients who have become addicted to AAS, as 15%–30% of users do, there is also the self-flagellation of personal failure, of weakness, because they were not able to cease use on their own due to the difficulty of withdrawal. Is their continuing use a case of "free choice, as many—including doctors—believe? I believe it is not. Not for those who are compelled to resume use by the overwhelming pain of withdrawal. For them, as for any other addict, their free will has been hijacked by their drug. The strong odds that this will happen to him or her must be understood by users. The unique nature of AAS addiction must be understood by policy makers and by physicians who are responsible to heal when addiction has occurred. Read more about this in Chapter 14 on AAS addiction and recovery.

I guess what I'm trying to say is that I know you all want to be monsters in the gym. I get that, but we must always (always!!) keep our health number one when we strive to achieve our physical goals. News of a lifter or bodybuilder dying from a condition related to their use of AAS is now frequent enough (two cases in just these past few weeks) to provide strong warnings. Are you thinking it happened to them because they used more than you, longer than you, had different genetics? Think again. There is no safe lane for AAS. There is always some risk. It's not cool dying when you're young… or having a heart attack at age 37. I have many patients at risk for this right now. Not long ago, a patient told me, "Doc, it was time for me to join up because I have had one heart attack and a quadruple bypass in the past 60 days." At age 44. This patient also said that many of his gym buddies from "back in the day" are either dead or have had heart attacks. There is, indeed, no free lunch in the weight room. Name your price.

So, what's the take-away? Gear down and, if you are on testosterone replacement therapy (TRT), stick with the lowest dose of physiological testosterone that you can. Hopefully you're diagnosed by a knowledgeable doctor. Also, make sure your cardiac risk factors are well managed: that means blood pressure, glucose, and lipids. I know I say it over and over again, but it's that important. All of the bad things I see in terms of heart disease and steroids are related to these basic medical risk factors. If men had perfect risk factor management, we would not see the scary things we do in the clinic. And, by the way, that is true for men, with or without steroid use or TRT. So if you're on steroids, get off and/or wean down under medical supervision with hormone replacement therapy (HRT) and treat the hell out of your risks! See your doctor and ask him or her to help you. Tell them they can give me a call, too.

8

Desperately
Seeking Adonis

I'm going to dive deep into the seas of the limbic brain (animal brain) of the lifter and discuss some of the basic origins of our drive to be "muscleheads." Sit back, enjoy our journey beneath the cerebral gray, and say hello to the amygdaloid nucleus. This is the region in our earliest limbic brain, the area responsible for our primitive drives and emotions—including hunger, aggression, fear, sex—that make up the root components of our personalities. As the lifter lifts—and lifts BIG—some of his satisfaction comes from satisfying limbic drives. As he meets his goals, he has an overall sense of well-being that satisfies other drives and needs. Perhaps he overcomes fear through being strong, or he feels his muscularity makes him more sexually attractive, for example. For some lifters, however, the satisfaction is short-lived. These are the lifters who become trapped in an endless, compulsively driven effort to attain what they believe, despite obvious gains, has not yet been achieved—their ideal body. When this lifter reacts by making choices that may actually be harmful, it suggests that their goal is not strength or appearance in and of themselves, but to satisfy a primitive drive, one which is never fully satisfied.

Because I care for their health, I'd like to understand the deeper

47

psychological forces that drive such lifters to excess. However, the clinical interaction does not typically offer me this opportunity. Each lifter should examine whether his choices reflect normal, mature goals —goals that do not prompt self-destructive behavior in the way that ungoverned primitive drives can. I'm not saying I don't love to be "bigger" myself, but when does this go beyond being a "normal" goal? Some clues are engaging in excessive exercising and having an unhealthy related lifestyle in an endlessly frustrating cycle to become bigger. This has been described as the Adonis complex (American Psychiatric Association, 2013).

Adonis and the Adonis Complex

Greek mythology tells a tale of Adonis, half man, half god, who was considered the ideal in male beauty. Conceived as a result of an incestuous relationship, he lived much of his short life in the Underworld, where he was manipulated by others and ultimately by his own narcissism. How does the Adonis complex, sometimes called "bigorexia," relate to men who lift excessively and are never satisfied with their results? Such lifters, obsessed with developing the "ideal" body, harbor a neurotic belief that they are not muscular enough to match this ideal, despite their actual large musculature. Their unrealistic body assessment is thought to be the result of a condition known as muscle dysmorphia, a specific form of body dysmorphia. Those who suffer from muscle dysmorphia tend to hold delusions that they are "skinny" or "too small," when they are actually often above-average in musculature. With this disorder, a person is preoccupied with thoughts concerning appearance, especially musculature. Muscle dysmorphia is fueled by selective attention to a perceived defect (too skinny body, underweight, etc.). Those with the disorder are hypervigilant to even small deviations from their perceived ideal body. Such individuals repeat negative and distorted self-statements concerning their appearance to such an extent that these become automatic reinforcing beliefs. As a result, muscle dysmorphia influences a person's mood, often causing depression or feelings of disgust, and causes constant comparing of their body to an unattainable ideal. Not infrequently, AAS are used to the extent that physical health is also seriously impaired.

Whether one describes this as an Adonis complex or any of its variants, it is undeniable that many men, and a growing number of women, are using AAS and training so intensely that their whole life revolves around training sessions and eating regimens, despite failing relationships, financial strains and endangered health.

Seeing so many desperate to lift BIG—despite significant social and health costs—and achieving only short-lived satisfaction from this has strengthened my belief in the potentially causative effect of muscle dysmorphia. When muscle dysmorphia is present, it is testimony to the power of an ungoverned limbic system to negatively influence behavior. The implication for passionate lifters is to govern their passion with reason, to understand them- selves and their goals, always mindful that their behaviors must respect their bodies, their minds, their lives.

References

American Psychiatric Association. *Diagnostic and statistical manual of mental disorders*, 5th ed. Arlington, VA: American Psychiatric Publishing, 2013

9

Muscle Dysmorphia:
Disease or Dedication?

*"I'm sure I have muscle dysmorphia. I
can't stop thinking I'm too small."*

*"I keep working out, hoping I'll reach a
point where I'm satisfied with how I look."*

*"I do get bigger, but it's never enough;
I still keep feeling small."*

*"I look in the mirror, and I like what I see. If this is a
medical condition, I'm glad I have it! Bigorexia,
Yes! It improves your health, your physique, your
self confidence."*

Muscle Dysmorphia? Bigorexia? Or
Healthy Muscle Building?

Is a mental health " condition" sending men and women to gyms

51

and supplement suppliers in such increasing numbers? Or is it simply a healthy quest for strength and the ideal in physical beauty? Is getting bigger, faster, and stronger the path to Nirvana? Or is it a neurotic quest that never leads to satisfaction and that, paradoxically, moves the goal farther away just as one achieves it? Endless frustration punctuated by interludes of exhilaration. At what point can seeking the perfect body turn on that same body— as well as the mind—hijacking both in an obsessive cycle? Or is it the other way around: Does a hijacked mind lead to a relentless and obsessive search for the "perfect" body? And, finally, why do these questions matter? Beyond being posted and parried in just about every blog and website devoted to muscle building and manipulated by the supplements manufacturers who fund these sites, these questions have become a serious topic in the world of medicine. (Pope et al, 2005)

Although muscle dysmorphia is currently diagnosed as a subset of body dysmorphia disorder, there is debate as to whether it can exist independent of body dysmorphia disorder .(Hitzroth et al, 2001; Pope et l, 2005) At present, clinicians use two specifiers to identify subgroups of body dysmorphic individuals to determine the presence of muscle dysmorphia:

Muscle Dysmorphia Specifiers

- Constantly examine themselves in a mirror
- Frequently compare themselves with others
- Hate their reflections
- Become distressed if they miss a workout session or one of their many meals a day
- Become distressed if they do not receive enough protein per day in their diet

- Take potentially dangerous anabolic steroids
- Neglect jobs, relationships, or family because of excessive exercising
- Have delusions of being underweight or below average in musculature.
- In extreme cases, inject appendages with fluid (for example, synthol)

- Insight Specifier:

  How convinced the individual is that his or her belief about appearance   of the disliked body parts is true ("I am ugly/too fat/too thin/deformed.") (American Psychiatric Association, 2013)

Most of the above behaviors are the professional concerns of psychiatrists and others in the mental health field. However, the effects of anabolic steroids—which figure prominently in extreme muscle building—should be of concern to all medical professionals.

AAS, Supplements and Muscle Dysmorphia

There is clearly a synergistic relationship between the phenomenal growth of the supplements industry and increased world-wide interest in muscle building. It has been apparent for some time that use of AAS is a required accelerant for extreme muscle building. (Epstein, 2015; Yesalis et al, 1993) Extreme muscle building has now moved well beyond the hard core bodybuilder and the professional athlete whose use is not for muscle building for its own sake, but to increase their chances of winning at their sport. Which of the many groups who depend on AAS now for extreme muscle building have muscle dysmorphia—"bigorexia"? Which simply have an intense and useful dedication to building the strongest, fastest, or most beautiful body possible? This is an ongoing debate that now also considers the question of the power of changing ideals and social and cultural norms about the ideal male body. Regarding this, I have to say that when I look at sculptures of the ideal male body as far back as the days of high Greek civilization, I find it hard to believe that muscularity wasn't always the ideal. Nothing terribly new there. Actually, it's the trendy slim Jim look that puzzles me. Oh, well, de gustibus…

These debates make great reading for those who enjoy going into the weeds, but here on the ground we now have enough empirical evidence that there is a point at which disease can be distinguished from dedication. Checklists such as the one cited earlier can be helpful to recognize when behavior has turned from healthy muscle building to harmful pathology.

Hypotheses about the underlying factors that drive the quest for extreme strength in the first place, and those that can cause it to morph from health to disease are still just that—hypotheses. However, the effects of crossing the divide from health to harm are observable and potentially treatable. For now, I will sidestep the definitional debate and simply continue to share what I have observed over years of treating men who love to train hard for better...and for worse.

References

American Psychiatric Association. *Diagnostic and statistical manual of mental disorders*, 5th ed. Arlington, VA: American Psychiatric Publishing, 2013

Brower, KJ. Anabolic androgenic steroid abuse and dependence in clinical practice, *Phys Sportsmed,* 2009;37(4):131-140

Epstein, D. Everyone's juicing, *Pro Publica*, Sept. 17, 2015

Hitzroth, V, Wessels, C, Zungu-Dirwayi, N, Oosthuizen, P, Stein, DJ. et al. Muscle dysmorphia: a South African sample, *Psychiatry Clin Neurosci,* 2001 Oct;55(5):521-523

Phillips, KA, Wilhelm, S, Koran, LM, Didie, ER, Fallon, BA, Feusner, J et al. Body dysmorphic disorder: some key issues for DSM-V, *Depress Anxiety,* 2010, Jun;27(6):573-591

Pope, HG, Menard, W, Fay, C, Olivardia, R, Phillips, KA. Clinical features of muscle dysmorphia among males with body dysmorphic disorder, *Body Image,* 2005 Dec;2(4):395-400

Pope, HG Jr, Gruber, AJ, Choi, P, Olivardia, R, Phillips, KA, Pope, HG et al. Muscle dysmorphia: an under-recognized form of body dysmorphic disorder, *Psychosomatics,* 1997, Nov-Dec;3860:548-557

Rahnema, C, Lipshultz, LI, Crosnoe, LE, Kovac, JR, Kim, ED. Anabolic steroid induced hypogonadism: diagnosis and treatment, *Fertil Steril,* 2014 May;101(5):1271-1279

Talih, F et al. Anabolic steroid abuse: psychiatric and physical costs, *Cleve Clin J Med,* 2007 May;74(5):341-352

Wood, RI. Anabolic-androgenic steroid dependence? *Front Neuroendocrinol,* 2009 Oct;29(4):490-506

Yesalis, CE, Kennedy, NJ, Kopstein, AN, Bahrke, MS. Anabolic-androgenic steroid use in the United States, *JAMA,* 1993 Sept 8;270(10):1217-1221

10

Roid Rage

Trying to understand "roid rage" is a frustrating undertaking— and not just for me. From the ambiguous findings of (usually) small studies, to sensational media accounts and passionate posts from roid deniers on steroid-user websites, it's clear that there is neither popular nor professional consensus on the definition of this phenomenon or what causes it. At this point, the best we can do is look at a representative sample of these sources and try to see what (if any) points of agreement there are.

I have read reams of professional literature on steroids and psychiatric events. Unfortunately, this only increased the confusion around the question. In most cases, reports on the relationship of AAS and roid rage concluded with some version of "We just don't know for sure." So, there's no slam dunk consensus on this issue. In 2010, Kanayama and colleagues summarized the state of the art of psychiatric effects of AAS:

"The consensus of the field studies is that some

AAS users exhibit hypomanic or manic symptoms during AAS exposure, occasionally (albeit rarely) accompanied by psychotic symptoms. Some studies have also reported users showing depressive symptoms, occasionally associated with suicide, usually during AAS withdrawal. However, it is impossible to estimate the prevalence of these syndromes in the overall population of illicit AAS users, because there is such wide variation among the various studies. Some studies report relatively frequent and often severe pathology (Pope and Katz, 1988; Thiblin et al., 1999b), whereas others find little or even none (Bahrke et al., 1992). These differences may be partially attributable to differences in the doses of AAS used, with more frequent symptoms in studies that included large numbers of high-dose AAS users (particularly those ingesting the equivalent of more than 1000 mg of testosterone per week." (Kanayama et al, 2010)

One thing I can definitely agree with is that when people take large doses of AAS and certain types of AAS, like tren (AKA Devil's juice), their personalities can change. No experienced steroid user will argue this. Unlike studies where there are clear measurable variables and end points (for example, blood pressure, lipid values, or kidney function), determining the specific cause-and-effect relationship between AAS use and psychiatric issues is onerously complex. For one thing, when defining roid rage, one has to consider the perspective of who is being questioned about it. When AAS users are asked about roid rage, they often get defensive and minimize its existence, whereas non-AAS users tend to accept out of hand that such a state co-exists with AAS use. And neither group seems able to provide adequate scientific support for its contention. (Kanayama et al, 2010) I have also found that researchers are careful to differentiate TRT from AAS use, and frank psychosis from impulse control. Nave and colleagues demonstrated that a single dose of testosterone increases the probability that a man will react intuitively rather than reflectively to stimuli (Nave et al, 2017). When I draw from my professional experiences, I would say that it is true that impulse control is a *psychiatric* feature that is affected by AAS use. However, I cannot say that there are definitive *behavioral* changes that occur secondary to AAS use—at least no changes that can be precisely quantified. It's also worth noting that, putting the issue in perspective, the accounts of damaging or harmful violent behavior correctly or incorrectly attributed to roid rage pale when one considers that there are millions of people actively using AAS.

So, we still can't say for sure that AAS-related impulse control regulation is truly pathologic. If so, is it reproducible with AAS use, and what are the processes underlying it? We simply don't have AAS data comparable to what we have on alcohol and other drugs (illicit or prescription)—or even caffeine—which would make it possible to confidently consider the contribution of AAS to aggressive behavior, poor impulse control, and even death. With agents like alcohol, caffeine, and nicotine that are permitted in American culture, we have developed an expectation of self-regulation and personal responsibility when it comes to dealing with their negative effects. Will AAS use and roid rage follow the same model? That remains to be seen. What I can tell you is this: People who use AAS know that they can experience occasional emotional lability, but for the most part, the great majority of AAS users experience a sense of well-being. For better or worse, it's one of the reasons they stay on these agents for extended periods. My take as a scientist is that that crazy guy on gear is just as likely to be an asshole—on steroids.

References

Kanayama, G, Hudson, JI, Pope, HG Jr. Illicit anabolic- androgenic steroid use, *Horm Behav*, 2010 June;58(1):111-121

Nave, G, Nadler, A, Zava, D, Camerer, C. Single-dose testosterone administration .... *Psychol Sci,* 2017 Oct. 28;(10):1398–1407

11

Is the Doctor In?

A number of AAS experts, including Dr. Shalender Bhasin, of Harvard University, have made clear the extent and seriousness of the burgeoning public health issue involving AAS users, and the ethical responsibility of physicians to meet this by informing themselves about AAS and treatment protocols that have been demonstrated to provide safe and effective symptom relief for AAS side effects and to support cessation. (Canavan, 2013) A recent systematic review of AAS research encompassing all AAS studies conducted between 1965 and 2013, including voluntary interviews with users, has provided a guide for what physicians will need to know and what AAS users should expect when they seek medical help. (Rahnema, 2014). Some of their recommendations are discussed in Chapter 31 on anabolic androgenic steroid–induced hypogonadism (ASIH).

Hopefully, wider dissemination of these recommendations will begin to change the clinical situation for AAS users who are experiencing the psychoendocrinal symptoms of AAS. Currently, too many users—as well as doctors—are unaware of the relationship between AAS use and these serious and potentially permanent effects. (Kovac et al, 2014) The lack of awareness among users is regularly demonstrated in online AAS forums, which reveal an alarming level of risk-taking in the substances users choose and the levels at which these are used. Expressions of regret for such choices are also found regularly on these websites.

While medical publications indicate some increase in involvement by physicians in the care of AAS users, 56% of users have never disclosed their use to doctors; most continue to be reluctant to seek professional medical help even for serious side effects, relying instead on information they find on the web and in the gym to guide them. (Pope and Brower, 2004) The poor reliability of this peer advice is demonstrated by the number of posts about serious and sometimes irreversible damage a user has sustained as a result of basing choices on something they read online. That is not to say that there are not competent advice givers posting online—usually more seasoned users—who demonstrate remarkably broad knowledge of AAS. These writers are also more likely to caution young men against beginning to use and to advise users with serious side effects to seek medical care.

Since getting reliable peer advice about AAS is clearly a hit-or-miss proposition, why do so many users continue to risk serious harm by relying on this resource? Why would a man who is experiencing severe loss of libido, unabating depression— hallmarks of ASIH—not seek a medical professional for help? Why would a man who wishes to stop using AAS, but is unable to do so on his own because of intolerable withdrawal symptoms, not seek medical help?

According to a 2004 study by Pope and Brower, some clues to their reluctance can be found on AAS peer websites: Exchanges between users reinforce disdain for doctors based on negative experiences with those they found to be uninformed about AAS, unempathic toward their suffering from

AAS side effects, and of little help with cessation beyond demands to "just stop using"— despite unbearable withdrawal symptoms.

Following up on previous studies of patient stigmatization by physicians, researchers at three major Northeast medical universities found that medical providers had a more negative perception of patients with AAS use or eating disorders than they had of either cocaine users or healthy adults. Thus, the authors concluded, addressing physician bias could help reduce both the personal suffering and the public health burden related to AAS use. (Yua et al, 2015) AAS users also report not seeking medical care or being open with their physicians because they fear that doctors might report them for using illegal substances. To remove these obstacles to providing and receiving appropriate medical help, the following are essential:

- Doctors must become knowledgeable about safe and effective treatment protocols for AAS side effects and for safe and effective cessation.

- Doctors must bring to the doctor-patient relationship unconditional regard for the patient, regardless of the doctor's personal feelings on anabolic steroid use.

- To receive the best medical care, patients need to be open with doctors about their use, what agents they have used, and for how long.

- Patients should inform themselves about, and determine whether their doctor also understands, the laws regulating confidentiality of their medical information.

For patients who are attempting to wean from AAS, experts have advised doctors to provide whatever medications and other measures are needed to support safe and effective withdrawal, providing these to a patient until normal hormonal levels are restored, monitoring treatment closely, and adjusting treatment until normal levels are restored. (Hochberg et al, 2003; Rahnema et al, 2014; Spratt, 2012; Talih et al, 2007; Zitzmann and Nieschlag, 2000) When normal levels are not restored, and permanent hypogonadal-pituitary-testicular damage is apparent, testosterone replacement therapy may need to be considered. Such protocols have been shown to help patients avoid the cycle of re-use which occurs when unsupported withdrawal becomes unbearable (Brower, 2009; Kanayama et al, 2015), and to prevent permanent hormonal damage that can occur when appropriate treatment is not provided in a timely manner. (Boregowda, 2011; Rahnema et al, 2014) As more physicians become familiar with the forego- ing recommendations, "cold turkey" treatments, which expose patients to distressing and potentially dangerous hormonal collapse, should eventually go the way of other unsupportable medical protocols of the past.

Just as it is the physician's professional responsibility to arm himself or herself with knowledge about the effects of AAS use, it is the user's personal responsibility to learn as much as he can about these agents. That is, to consult reliable sources of information about the makeup of any of the powerful agents he is thinking about using and the potential risks associated with this choice. The short-term side effects of using AAS become evident very soon. Self-treating to counteract these may provide cover for a while, but as the Anabolic Doc has been preaching, "There is no free lunch". (O'Connor, 2012) Taming the effects of powerful drugs by using equally powerful drugs, guided by Internet recipes, is a risky brew. Too often, as I have written previously here and elsewhere, the tragic paradoxical result is serious long-lasting or even permanent harm to the body on which so much time, money, and effort has been invested.

If a user decides to seek medical help for his symptoms or to help him wean safely and effectively, how can he determine whether his physician has adequate knowledge, empathy, and availability to partner with him on his journey back to health? As with most other important partnerships in life, the direct approach is the one most likely to yield the most information and, as a result, the best outcome. This approach requires the patient to be open about his use: what agents were used; for how long; and the effects of these on his body, mind, and relationships. The patient should directly inquire about how much the physician knows about AAS and its side effects, and determine how interested the physician seems to be in helping him. Both patient and doctor should recognize that treating the psychoendocrinological side effects of AAS, particularly ASIH, *requires timely medical intervention and close monitoring of the patient throughout treatment,* since patient response to treatment is very individual. The implication of this is frequent, regular contact with your physician until health is restored. Difficulty getting appointments should be a warning sign that doesn't bode well for a successful positive outcome.

A final word: Judgments about a patient's choice to use AAS have no place in the professional relationship. Medical advice, yes; judgments, no. If a physician does not seem to be well informed about AAS and its serious side effects, and if he or she doesn't seem open to a true partnership, or isn't sufficiently available to provide timely treatment monitoring, it's worth seeking another physician.

References

Boregowda, K, Joels, L, Stephens, JW, Price, DE. Persistent primary hypogonadism associated with anabolic steroid abuse. *Fertil Steril,* 2011 Jul;96(1):e7-8

Brower, KJ. Anabolic androgenic steroid abuse and dependence in clinical practice, *Physician Sportsmed,* 2009;37:131-140

Canavan, N. Endocrine society pumped up to raise steroid-abuse awareness, *Medscape,* December 17, 2013, http://www.medscape.com/viewarticle/817960

Hochberg, Z, Pacak, K, Chrousos, GP. Endocrine withdrawal syndromes, *Endocrine Rev,* 2003 Aug;24(4):523-534

Kanayama, G , Hudson, JI, DeLuca, J, Isaacs, S, Baggish, A, Weiner, R, Bhasin, S, Pope, HG Jr. Prolonged hypogonadism in males following withdrawal from anabolic androgenic steroids: an under-recognized problem, 2015 May;110(5):828-831. https://www.ncbi.nlm.nih.gov/pmc/articles/PMC4398624/

Kovac, JR et al. Men regret anabolic steroid use due to a lack of comprehension regarding the consequences on future fertility, *Andrologia,* http://onlinelibrary.wiley.com/doi/10.1111/ and.12340/abstract

O'Connor, T. No free lunch, *Muscular Development,* March 2012

Pope G, Brower, KJ. Treatment of anabolic-androgenic steroid related disorders. Chapter 17, in *The American Psychiatric Publishing textbook of substance abuse treatment,* eds. M. Galanter, H. Kleber, 2008

Rahnema, C et al. Anabolic steroid induced hypogonadism: diagnosis and treatment, *Fertil Steril,* 2014 May;101(5):1271- 1279

Spratt, D. Considering tapering testosterone replacement in certain patients, *Endocr Rev,* September 2014

Talih, F, Fattal, O, Malone, D Jr. Anabolic steroid abuse: psychiatric and physical costs, *Cleve Clin J Med,* 2007 May;74(5):341- 344, 346, 349-352

Yua, J et al. Healthcare professionals' stigmatization of men with anabolic androgenic steroid use and eating disorders, *ScienceDirect*, June 2015

Zitzmann, M, Nieschlag, E. Hormone substitution in male hypogonadism, *Mol Cell Endocrinol*, 2000 Mar 30;161(1-2): 73-88

12

Understanding the Strength Athlete: HardcoreMedicine

D ear Doctor,

Testimony to the universal quest for strength pre-dates modern society. One ancient legend tells us that a Greek wrestler, Milo of Croton, trained by carrying a newborn calf on his back every day until it was fully grown. And the Greek physician Galen described strength training exercises using the halteres, an early form of dumbbells, as early as the 2nd century. We've come a long way from the calf-carry, but the quest for strength persists. One wonders what the ancients would think of the super-human feats of strength we witness now! Even as recently as 20 years ago, people would have marveled at the feats of strength one can see every day in our gyms. The average "strong guy/gal in the gym today would have been a world record holder then. What we are seeing now has occurred secondary to dramatic improvements in training, gear, equipment, regimens, and of course supplements. I call these athletes who have dedicated their lives to serious training in the disciplines of powerlifting, bodybuilding, and strong man, "strength athletes." Never before have we seen such an explosion in the number of people engaged in these activities at all levels of participation, from the hobbyist to the professional. These athletes have taken their place in the sports world as examples of the limits of strength that can be attained by the human body.

The strength athlete lives—and thrives—by battling the forces of nature. Like any other activity, hardcore training regimens and lifestyles are governed by the basic laws of physics, including Newton's third law of motion: For every action, there is an equal and opposite reaction. The implications for the strength athlete are the many consequences of the intense biologic stress required for optimal performance levels. Thus, specialized medical care requires physicians to understand these stressors and their consequences, and to respect the person who has chosen to undergo these. In the case of the strength athlete, the latter includes respecting the unique lifestyle of these men and women while educating and treating them. Judging by the reluctance of strength athletes to consult with doctors, these requisites for compassionate and knowledgeable medical care are seen by them as lacking in too many physicians. The disconnect is even greater when these athletes have chosen to use steroids. A still too large number of physicians have, because of their lack of knowledge and/or their perceived personal bias against strength athletes, become untrusted by this population. As a result, though more than half of all strength athletes say they would like to see physicians for issues related to their sport, they are reluctant to do so. The majority report that even when they are experiencing symptoms, they avoid doctors whom they consider at best unknowledgeable and at worst judgmental. (Cohen et al, 2007) Thus, it would appear that unconditional acceptance of strength athletes by physicians is perceived as more the exception than the rule—especially when steroids use is suspected. But even use is not an issue, typical encounters are often described as having judgmental overtones, with the strength athlete seen as someone who has harmed himself unnecessarily. Additionally, concerns on the part of either physician or patient regarding the confidentiality of the medical encounter can negatively affect the strength athlete's medical care. For example, when the use of illegal substances is suspected or actual, critical patient data related to AAS may not be sought (by physician) or made available (by athlete). It should be clearly understood by both physician and patient that the law protects the confidentiality of their medical encounter in the same way it does any patient's.

The suffering of someone who has gone to extraordinary lengths to become strong, and whose appearance indicates extraordinary strength, may not elicit the sympathy which other patients bring forth, but a physician is not called to be sympathetic; he or she must maintain unconditional empathic and professional regard for all patients. It is concerning to hear or read about physicians who have reacted to these patients' requests for help with some version of "It's your own fault" regarding their symptoms, or their AAS dependency. (Yua et al, 2015) Only 2 years ago, a major medical journal published an article in which a physician reported recommending what amounted to going cold turkey, a "just say no" approach, when a patient who was suffering in withdrawal asked for help to end his use of AAS. This is totally unacceptable when there are safe, effective weaning protocols available to support cessation. It is clear that both the knowledge gap and the weak dissemination of available knowledge have been significant obstacles to appropriate medical care for strength athletes.

Beyond the obvious professional disservice when a patient is stigmatized in the clinical setting, a poor fit between doctors and strength athletes may also have contributed to missed opportunities to investigate the many health issues related to this sport. Additionally, encounters between physicians and strength athletes present valuable opportunities to investigate *in vivo* the mechanisms of action and the potentials and limits of human strength, and how they can be enhanced. Such learning from our strength athletes' experiences would benefit other populations whose full participation in

71

society may be compromised by their mobility and strength limitations due to muscle wasting diseases and even the aging process itself, for example. The enthusiasm and support of a number of medical colleagues who have indicated interest in learning more about treating the strength athlete validates again for me why I have chosen this profession. (Dobs, 1999) As I close this chapter, I realize that the knowledge and care of the strength athlete is not simply "hardcore" medicine; it is at the core of medicine itself.

References

Cohen, J et al. A league of their own..., *J Int Soc Sports Nutr*, 2007;4:12

Dobs, AS. Is there a role for androgenic anabolic steroids in medical practice? *JAMA*, Apr 14, 1999, 281(14):1326-1327

Yua, J et al. Healthcare professionals' stigmatization of men with anabolic androgenic steroid use and eating disorders, *Science Direct*, June 2015

13

Anabolic Androgenic Steroid-Induced Hypogonadism:

Why Men Can't Quit

Anabolic steroids, they will build you up…and take you down.

Official estimates indicate that the number of AAS users has tripled from one million to three million since these agents were declared illegal in the US in 1991. Independent experts, however, believe the number to be at least 4 million. And contrary to what you might think, based on media reports of AAS use by professional athletes, the largest groups of AAS users are not professional athletes but average men, women, and teens who do not compete in any sport. Of these users, 75% state that their use is for purely cosmetic reasons, primarily to achieve a lean and muscular physique. (Pope et al, 2014)

The development of AAS products, including at least 100 synthetic relatives of testosterone and a reported 15% to 25% of AAS-contaminated dietary supplements (advertised as AAS-free) has made it possible to enhance attempts to create their ideal body—to promote leanness and increase muscle mass and strength, while decreasing recovery time and improving healing. (Pope and Brower, 2008). However, as their hyphenated description indicates, *anabolic-androgenic steroids* aren't only anabolic (muscle building). Users must also contend with their androgenic (male sex hormones) effects. Thus, there have been many attempts to pharmacologically dissociate the desired anabolic actions of AAS from the unwanted androgenic side effects— especially those accompanying high doses of these agents. (Langenbucher et al, 2004)

Some of these androgenic side effects include serious liver damage (hepatotoxicity); bile blockage (cholestasis); renal kidney failure; inhibition of reproductive function, e.g., low sperm count or infertility (oligospermia/ azoospermia); and decreased production of natural testosterone (hypogonadism), leading to poor libido and lability in mood, acne, hair loss, and gynecomastia—physical feminization of males (e.g., breast swelling) which, when severe, can require surgery. (Langenbucher et al, 2004; Sullivan, in Kuhn, 2010; Rahnema et al, 2015)

Some of these side effects of AAS may be transient, resolving when AAS use is ended. However, they can also cause long-lasting or permanent end organ damage .(Rahnema et al, 2015) For example, high doses of AAS, used over long periods of time, have been shown to have long-lasting effects on the cardiovascular system, causing damage to the heart and blood vessels. (Baggish et al, 2017) Such cardiovascular effects can be seen in bodybuilders who typically use AAS in doses up to *one hundred times greater than the normal body amount*, risking clumping platelets in the heart and potentially triggering strokes and heart attacks. Even after stopping AAS, there may be a decrease in left ventricular function, leading to heart failure. (Sullivan, in Kuhn,

2002) I discuss these myriad effects in greater depth in other chapters. In this chapter, I will discuss the condition believed to be *universal in AAS users,* and the main reason why men who have used AAS come to see physicians. Anabolic steroid–induced hypogonadism (ASIH), a unique form of androgen deficiency denoting the shutting down of the hypothalamic pituitary/testicular (HPT) system due to AAS use. (Canavan, 2013)

ASIH: A Unique Hypogonadism

Recognized as the result of a complex and global endocrine disruption that accompanies long-term AAS use, including stacking (use of several AAS products simultaneously), cycling (on-and-off AAS use, typically over 12 weeks), and multiple high doses of ancillary drugs, ASIH has been well described in studies for at least a decade. (Kashkin & Kleber, 1989; Hochberg et al, 2003; Tan & Scally, 2009; Rahnema et al, 2014) Despite this, inadequate understanding by many physicians about ASIH or the drugs that cause it has contributed to underserving the AAS-using population—especially those who wish to cease using.

Noting that because ASIH is a unique and complex form of hypogonadism, Rahnema and colleagues caution that the "unique pharmacological milieu" resulting from long-term AAS use is such that "medical testosterone… which is given for testosterone replacement therapy (TRT), at a fixed replacement dose, may not be a good model to describe the pharmacodynamics of AAS". In their systematic review of AAS, based on interviews with hypogonadal users as well as research studies and clinical reports between 1965 and 2013, these authors have provided valuable insight into what is now known about ASIH and about protocols for safe and effective evidence-based treatments. Because such systematic reviews are based on the best available evidence, this comprehensive review is especially important to counteract the inaccurate—and even judgmental—ideas that may have influenced doctors' under-treatment of AAS users.

As a physician who has spent years researching medical issues related to AAS in both the ivory tower and the iron gym, I have had the good fortune to treat thousands of men who are completely open with me about their use. For 90% of these men who seek help regarding a health issue related to AAS, there is something related to sex in their motivation. It's guaranteed that, after years of AAS use, a man's testosterone will be low, and in most cases this individual will have a lower symptom threshold— for example, his poor libido will be more severe than that in a man with "organic" low testosterone. (Kelleher, 2004) The reason for this difference is unknown. However, we do know that prolonged periods of injecting esters of testosterone in high doses— higher than those used in standard testosterone replacement—leads to chronic higher free testosterone levels in the central nervous system (CNS). These chronic high levels of free testosterone cause changes in parts of the CNS, which may lead to dependency on superphysiologic testosterone doses for optimal sexual experience. "Chronically consumed high doses of AAS are postulated to stimulate brain reward systems in humans, and to result in neuroadaptations in other brain systems that manifest as withdrawal symptoms (e.g., poor libido) upon discontinuation". (Wood, 2004) That is, it is possible that long-term use, which causes permanent damage in these areas, contributes to severe low libido states when AAS are stopped. (Kanayama et al, 2015)

When the Music Stops

Men, even young men with normal testosterone levels, experience increased libido when they are on AAS. However, the operant word here is "on". As any experienced steroid AAS user quickly learns, sex "on" steroids vs "off" is very different. In the beginning, most steroid AAS users, whether or not they use post cycle therapy (PCT) to counteract the androgenic effects of AAS, experience only minimal sexual side effects. However, whether a user is cycling or attempting to permanently cease using, the hypogonadal state during withdrawal from AAS can cause poor libido, impotence, infertility, severe depression, and even suicidality. (Brower, 2009; Kanayama et al, 2015)

To try to understand the relationship between AAS and the sexual issues that are prevalent in ASIH, we must understand the dynamics of some of the most widely used agents. In addition to a variety of testosterone-based agents (for example, testosterone cypionate, enanthate, propionate), there are testosterone-derived drugs like Dianabol and boldenone. There are also dihydrotestos- terone (DHT)–derived agents like Anadrol and Anavar, and the 19-nortestosterone (19-nor) AAS agents like Deca-Durabolin and Trenbolone. (Web MD, 2013) Each of these agents has specific chemical effects that affect a man's sexual function. However, they all share one effect which is mediated by the HPT system: They will ALL shut down a man's natural testosterone production while he is taking the drug. Specific drugs, doses, and individual user profile will influence the severity of this inevitable hypogonadal outcome. For example, drugs like trenbolone and Deca-Durabolin are known to be very suppressive to the HPT system—hence, the classic term since the 1970s, "Deca-dick.

The method of action (MOA) for this severe shutdown may be related not only to the suppression of endogenous testosterone, but also to the fact that Deca-Durabolin is reduced to dihydronandrolone (DHN) as opposed to DHT which, along with endogenous testosterone, binds with androgen receptors in the brain to support libido in naturally intact males. When DHN then crosses the blood-brain barrier, interacting with androgen receptors in the brain, it may either compete with DHT and testosterone or act as a direct antagonist, causing inhibitory actions and resulting in a low libido state. We also know that 19-nor drugs like Deca-Durabolin and trenbolone, which are synthetic progestins, can cause increased prolactin production which can lead to diminished libido and non-optimal CNS dopaminergic states.

A popular "bro science" remedy for this low libido state— widely published on AAS websites and forums—is to take greater parts of testosterone-to-nandrolone doses; most experienced users recommend a 1.5 to 2:1 ratio. And men say this works— for a time. Men almost never take a nandrolone agent like Deca or Tren without testosterone. And when they are on these drugs, sexual performance is usually not only preserved, but most men say they are hypersexual during this time. It appears that the combination of a 19-nor drug and testosterone esters provides overstimulation to the sexual areas of the brain. Again, for a period of time. Then things can come crashing down! The

CNS, which is dynamic, always in flux, tries to maintain balance in reaction to continuous stimulation, and makes adjustments to, among other things, various and changing hormone levels and chemistry(s). Thus, though AAS provides an initial stimulation of the androgen receptors in the brain that results in a libido upswing, it can also cause permanent damage in these and other areas, contributing to severe low libido states when AAS are stopped. (Kanayama et al, 2015)

In addition to suppressing the HPT system, AAS use causes imbalances that affect the sex-related levels of hormones (including estrogen, androgen, prolactin—as discussed above in the case of the nandrolone-based AAS—and DHT) and CNS neurotransmitters (such as serotonin, dopamine, norepinephrine, and GABA–gamma-aminobutyric acid). "The potential variability of molecular and cellular effects of the AAS in the brain suggest that the range of actions of these steroids will be highly complex, depending not only upon the chemical signatures and concentrations of the different AAS taken, but also upon region-specific differences in AR (androgen receptors) ERα, ERβ, and aromatase expression and changes in the endogenous steroid environment that occur as a function of sex, age and hormonal state". (Penatti et al, 2011)

I have seen evidence of the complexity of the relationship between steroid use and sexual side effects in the thousands of interviews I have had with men who use AAS and/or those who are on TRT. When I attempted to assess their sexual response to these agents, I was amazed at the variability, and at their sometimes paradoxical responses. Some men told me that they feel best on 1,500 mg of AAS a week, whereas others receiving TRT reported that just 2 days after a physiologic replacement dose of 100 mg testosterone cypionate, their libido is poor, and they feel best just prior to the next injection nadir. Clearly, sexual response to these agents is no simple formula.

Many men who use AAS chronically also use a drug called Dostinex (Web MD, 2013) to block the effects of elevated prolactin levels secondary to AAS, and to improve libido. However, the side effects of this drug, which is a dopamine promoter used to treat certain hormonal or hyperprolactinemic disorders either from unknown medical conditions or from pituitary growths, can be serious and can lead to other medical problems, such as low blood pressure, nausea, vomiting, shortness of breath, ankle swelling, fertility issues, and severe mood disorders. A drug for a drug, for yet another drug? Is it worth it?

In my clinical practice, I have also observed that men taking AAS—or even on physiologic testosterone—have poor erections at times, despite a perfectly balanced hormonal milieu. In a 2015 study, Kanayama and colleagues found that a subset of AAS users treated for ASIH showed continued loss of sexual desire and erectile dysfunction even when normal testosterone levels were restored. The authors concluded that, "Such cases may possibly represent end organ resistance—reflecting a possibly irreversible down-regulation of androgen receptors or androgen receptor signaling mechanisms." Since almost 100% of men on chronic AAS and TRT have atrophied testicles and thus experience a venous leak state, they can experience poor-quality erections. A urologist colleague explained it to me like this: "The testicles are like dampers at the base of the penis. When the testicle is shrunken and atrophied, the ability to hold back blood in the erect engorged penis may be reduced, leading to a leak-like situation and poor sustained quality erections."

Withdrawal Syndrome

Inseparable from the issue of ASIH is what happens when a man comes off AAS, either during cycling or in a cessation attempt. For most men, being on AAS leads to either great sex or none— or at least difficulty having sex. But remember: The specific user hormonal profile, as well as the type, combinations, and doses of AAS and any ancillary drugs that are being taken, play a role in one's sexual experience on AAS. It's when a man *stops* using AAS that everything falls apart—regardless of what agents were used. The common denominator then is ASIH. This is what the average user does not know or understand…or consider when making the choice to use.

So, what exactly is going on here? The HPT system, which has been dormant while on AAS, has to start back up again when AAS is removed from the system. This takes time, and for men who have been on AAS for prolonged periods or used high doses and/or very suppressive AAS, the restoration of the HPT system is uncertain. It may take months or years—or, as noted earlier, the restoration may never occur, even with medical intervention. (Rahnema et al, 2014; Kanayama et al, 2015).

The most distressing withdrawal symptoms—impotence, poor libido, depression, and suicidality—can be so severe as to create a state of dependency in users who then feel compelled to resume use. When severe, withdrawal symptoms caused by ASIH can compromise attempts to end AAS and have also been shown to cause the palliative use of other illegal substances—for example, opiates. (Kanayama and Brower et al, 2010) The gravest danger during the AAS withdrawal period is severe depression and suicidality: 12% of users in withdrawal experience severe depression, and 5% attempt suicide. (Brower, 2009) It is not only the severity of withdrawal symptoms (particularly depressed libido and mood) but also just the *fear* of having these symptoms that can compel reuse and thus entrench the cycle of dependency. (Brower, 2009; Rahnema et al, 2014)   Dependency is believed to occur in 15% to 30% of AAS users (Kanayama & Brower et al, 2009), with AAS considered to be more addictive than cocaine. (Phillips, 2010) Because of these high rates of dependence, several experts proposed including AAS among the addictive or dependent substances in the Diagnostic and Statistical Manual of Mental Disorders. (Kanayama et al, 2009) The take-home message here is that withdrawal syndrome is the MOST COMMON REASON WHY MEN DO NOT AND CANNOT STOP USING STEROIDS; why they are compelled to stay on steroids for prolonged periods, and even for life.

Post Cycle Therapy

The pathophysiology of AAS withdrawal is not fully understood. It may relate to the fact that during AAS use, the hypothalamus and pituitary go into a dormant state called apoptosis (programmed cell death) so that their production of gonadotropins—luteinizing hormone (LH) and follicle-stimulating hormone (FSH)—is inadequate to produce sustained testicular testosterone. (Kanayama et al, 2008)   To counter this, AAS users have turned to a treatment protocol called post cycle therapy (PCT) in an attempt to hasten the restoration of the HPT and to minimize the devastating physiological and psychological effects of ASIH in the post-use period.

The medical agents used for PCT are fertility medications of the class known as selective estrogen receptor modulators (SERMs), e.g., tamoxifen and Clomid, human chorionic gonadotropin (HCG), and various anti-estrogen medications (for example, Arimidex and letrozole). There is impressive support from experts for the medical use of these agents to support cessation by ameliorating withdrawal symptoms during treatment focused on restoring the HPT system and production of endogenous testosterone .(Hochberg et al, 2003; Pope and Brower, 2008; Rahnema et al, 2014; Spratt, 2012; Talih et al, 2007) However, it should be stated that although it is ethical for a physician to use these agents to assist any man coming off AAS, neither medical nor various other PCT regimens have been shown to produce sustainable endogenous testosterone levels or quality libido states in men who have used AAS chronically. I have had a number of patients who have used AAS say to me, "Doc, I did my PCT, but now I feel terrible and my testosterone and sex is down! What happened? Why didn't the PCT work?" The answer is, we just don't know. The following comment about PCT, which appeared on a popular Internet anabolic steroids blog, indicates the persistence of an overly optimistic view of the pathway back to normal following AAS use:

> *"Once the use of the AAS is complete and all of the exogenous steroidal hormones have cleared your system, natural testosterone recovery will begin again. Natural recovery assumes no prior low testosterone condition. It also assumes no damage was done to the HPTA (HPT) due to improper AAS use [emphasis added]. While natural recovery will occur on its own, it will be slow.*

For this reason, most are encouraged to implement a PCT plan after AAS use. Such a plan will commonly include the SERM's Nolvadex and Clomid, and often additional HCG. This will greatly speed up the recovery process, as well as its overall efficiency. It will not return your natural testosterone levels to normal on its own. If this is something you've been told, [(know that)] it is a myth. However, it will ensure you have testosterone for proper bodily function while your levels continue to naturally rise. Total recovery will still take months, but this will cut the total time down dramatically and ensure a smooth recovery."

"Total recovery; a smooth recovery"? Very comforting words, but such views should stress more emphatically what we now know about the potentially ravaging long-term and even permanent effects of ASIH in patients suffering the consequences of long-term, high-dose AAS use. It's important to discourage overly sanguine assurances about an automatic restart button after AAS use, especially since a significant number of high school students—the fastest-growing group of users—do not believe that these agents are harmful. (DOJ, 2004; Partnership for Drug- Free Kids, 2016)

ASIH: Threat to Cessation

Although the processes underlying AAS dependency/addiction are not yet fully understood, similarities to opioid addiction have been reported. (Wood, 2004; Caraci et al, 2011) Sexual and other physiological symptoms of withdrawal, e.g., flu-like symptoms, low mood, whether in cycling or in attempts to end use, were described some time ago by experts who noted that these were probably an endocrine effect of the episodic nature of use and discontinuance (cycling). (Kashkin and Kleben, 1989; Hochberg et al, 2003) A component part of the explanation of dependency, is the psychological explanation that when steroid use stops, muscle development is limited, and related feelings of power and self-esteem are impacted. Co-morbid conditions such as pre-existing depression and body dysmorphia are also thought to contribute to dependency. (Leone et al, 2005) This complex symptom profile causes AAS dependency to differ significantly from that of other addictive drugs, which are valued primarily for the "high" they produce. Thus, it is clear that education— though it is an important component in prevention efforts, as with other addictive drugs—is not sufficient for safe and effective AAS withdrawal when a man is seeking AAS cessation, any more than it would be for opioid or heroin withdrawal.

This complex and well-characterized AAS withdrawal syndrome has now been described as a major physiological factor in the development of AAS dependence, which has been called the most intractable of all substance abuse due to its dysphoric withdrawal effects which often lead to resumption of AAS use for relief. (Kanayama, Brower et al, 2009; Bhasin et al, 2011; Brower, 2009) As Brower noted in a 2009 article, the physiological nature of dependency on AAS can be diagnosed by asking what happens when a patient tries to stop using AAS. Thus, he cautions that, "Conventional methods of treating substance abuse are usually inappropriate unless modified specifically for AAS users." Despite such warnings, treatment for AAS dependence continues to be modeled after other treatments for dependence on other substances. (See Chapter 14 on AAS and addiction.)

Because of the unique pathophysiology of ASIH which distinguishes hypogonadal AAS users from other substance abusers, as well as from other hypogonadal populations, treatment protocols used by physicians familiar with AAS differ significantly from those used by physicians who are not as informed. Informed physicians recognize that safe and effective withdrawal from AAS should be supported by hormonal replacement therapy, tapering hormones down over time, and continuing until the HPT axis recovers. Recommended management strategies include TRT, human chorionic gonadotropin (hCG), and SERMs to restore the HPT axis and its ability to produce endogenous testosterone. (Hochberg et al, 2003; McBride et al, 2015; Pope and Brower, 2008; Rahnema et al, 2014; Spratt, 2012; Talih et al, 2007) Response to treatment will depend on damage done to the HPT during use.

(Boregowda et al, 2011; Kanayama et al, 2010)   Failure to provide timely appropriate treatment for ASIH could result in permanently failed HPT axis. (Rahnema et al, 2014)

Medications such as those listed above to relieve withdrawal symptoms and assist HPT recovery have been found to be both effective and safe in physiologic doses. McLaren et al (2012) found that short-term (up to 5 years). TRT has been found to result in minimal prostatic growth or development of lower urinary tract obstructive symptoms.

When AAS Requires Long Term TRT

Almost all AAS-related sexual issues will be related to libido. I find it puzzling that so many doctors give AAS users Viagra for their sexual issues, when it is largely useless! An AAS user's poor libido is not a failure of the man's penis to produce nitric oxide. In most cases, a user's poor libido will be the result of ASIH, as his CNS has adapted to higher levels of androgen while on AAS. As discussed above, the HPT is the main player here, and even with PCT, the shortest amount of time a man can expect to gain full restoration of the HPT is 3 to 6 months. If he still has a poor libido at that point he should consider the possibility of more severe ASIH and seek further medical evaluation and treatment.

SERMs such as those mentioned earlier may help a man experiencing AAS-related sexual issues. However, if these do not work, life-long physiologic TRT may have to be considered—a significant treatment choice whose seriousness cannot be overstated.

Life-long TRT involves considerable expense and inconvenience, and it also has potential implications for cardiovascular and prostate health, among other medical concerns. These are also discussed in Chapter 27, "Challenges to Personalizing Testosterone Replacement Therapy with the AAS User."

Cardiovascular Disease and AAS

The relationship of testosterone to heart disease is complex and multifactorial, but very real! Focusing on this is an important part of TRT treatment. AAS (including testosterone) have been shown to worsen existing heart disease risk factors such as hypertension and poor lipid ratios (higher LDL and low HDL), and to cause obstructive sleep apnea, which can lead an enlarged heart and heart failure. Other risks include increasing red blood cell counts, hypercoagulable states, and direct adverse effect on the heart muscle itself (cardiomyopathy) and to the endothelial aspect of the arteries, leading to plaque progression and the potential for a heart attack. (Morgentaler and Conners, 2015)

Since beginning my medical practice in 2005, I have seen many men with heart disease secondary to AAS use. This disease state can take decades to progress, and men with poor family histories associated with early and severe heart disease are especially at risk. Identifying these risk factors early is very important because, in addition to supporting safe and effective AAS discontinuation, physicians can play an important role in providing protective medicines while someone is going through a dangerous period of use. Treating hypertension, lipid abnormalities, polycythemia, sleep apnea, and other medical issues related to AAS use is the ethical thing to do, and informed physicians will do this. However, even now it is recognized that while long-term AAS use is associated with myocardial dysfunction and accelerated coronary atherosclerosis, the prevalence of these effects in AAS users continues to be an under-recognized public health problem. (Baggish et al, 2017) Give a man time to make the right decision, and prevent him from having a heart attack, has always been my perspective.

Prostate Disease

The debate continues about the connection between prostate disease and the cumulative effects of long-term testosterone treatment. Following an FDA warning on this issue, in 2016, Nam and Wallis presented their findings from a study of over 38,000 men, both treated and untreated. They found no increase in prostate risk in men who were treated for at least 5 years; the authors also found that risk actually decreased with long-term exposure. However, the design of the study has been criticized by other experts, who continue to advise caution. Because there are no long-term studies of men on testosterone treatment, it is reasonable to exercise caution in providing testosterone treatment of men with a family history of prostate disease or pre-existing malignancy. Current recommendations are to exclude prostate cancer before initiating TRT in men over age 40 and to closely monitor men in the first year of testosterone replacement, followed by observation in subsequent years. (Barqawi and Crawford, 2006)

In the chapter, "Personalizing TRT with the AAS User," I discuss many considerations that apply to both AAS users and non-using hypogonadal men. What must be stressed is that when a man's hypogonadism is AAS related, physicians must be able to interpret signs and symptoms of hypogonadism *in the context of AAS use,* and not simply apply guidelines that were developed for hypogonadal men in general. For example, because of the multi-system side effects of AAS use, as well as its unique pathophysiology, and the added complication of patient-specific use patterns, it is important for physicians to ask patients directly about their use in order to provide appropriate treatment and to counsel about cessation. Failure to ask patients directly about use can lead to misidentifying the underlying cause of many health problems, including hypogonadism and infertility.

Asking about AAS use should be part of the routine medical workup of all hypogonadal men. Specific questions should include: dates of first and last use; the names and doses of AAS used; sources of drugs (legal or prescription); routes of administration (including, for example, needle sharing); and patterns of use (e.g., stacking, cycling). Also of interest should be other drug combinations, for example those used to augment AAS effect: human growth hormone (HCG), insulin, selective androgen receptor modulators (SARMs), peptides, and clenbuterol; and drugs used to reduce unwanted side effects, for example, in post cycle therapy (PCT): Clomid, HCG, tamoxifen, and various anti-estrogens); and also drugs used to mask urine testing (e.g.,probenecid, diuretics). Doctors should also ask about the use of other illicit drugs such as opioids or heroin. (Pope and Brower, 2008)

AAS and Infertility

When physicians do not inquire about AAS use in cases of infertility—despite the fact that male infertility has been linked to prior or current steroid use—a couple may be unnecessarily led into an expensive and potentially frustrating course(s) of fertility treatment. AAS-related male infertility, which can sometimes be long-term, or even irreversible, has also caused a significant number of men who have used AAS to later express regret because they had not known that elevated serum testosterone levels obtained from AAS result in oligospermia and azoospermia. (Kovac et al, 2015) It's not clear that most physicians are aware of this either, or of the fact that the main cause of severe hypogonadism in young men is previous AAS use. (Crosnoe-Shipley et al, 2015)

A database study of 6,033 men of varying ages who sought treatment for hypogonadism from 2005 to 2010 found that prior anabolic steroid use is common in young men who seek treatment for hypogonadism, with hypogonadal men younger than 50 years being more than 10 times more likely to have prior AAS exposure than men 50 years or older. Further, in men with profound hypogonadism, AAS use was the most common etiology. (Coward et al, 2013) These findings add to a growing body of knowledge which makes it clear that it is time to review the medical profession's approach to evaluation and treatment of hypogonadism which has heretofore been focused on aging men.

Physicians Begin to Meet the Challenge

In the Endocrine Society's 2010 clinical guidelines on treating hypogonadism, neither AAS nor ASIH were mentioned in either the text, references, or illustrative tables. However, in 2013, an Endocrine Society expert panel was convened, presumably to address this deficit. The expert panel's final report issued a call for physicians to become better informed about AAS and related conditions like ASIH, to understand and respond to the motivations of users in a non-judgmental way, and to study the mechanisms of action of AAS. Despite the panel's acknowledgment that there is much yet to discover about the effects of AAS, it was noted that the one side effect that is "nearly universal" in users is the suppression of testicular function—ASIH. (Canavan, 2013) ASIH has been referred to as *the only substance abuse disorder worldwide which has not been adequately studied*, but with more AAS research being published and disseminated to physicians, we should be seeing a new day for appropriate medical care for millions of men—of all ages—currently suffering from, or at risk for, ASIH. As knowledgeable and caring partners, physicians will also be able to reverse their image as being reluctant to treat AAS users (Kanayama and Brower, 2010) and, as a result, also play a crucial role in prevention.

Valid and Timely Diagnosis

Targeted treatment of ASIH must begin with a valid diagnosis— that is to say, one that is informed by the distinct characteristics of this unique form of hypogonadism. In a 2009 article, Brower's operational definition for diagnosis of ASIH—"To confirm the physiological basis of dependence (on AAS), just ask the patient how he feels when he stops use"—is based on the fact that, over time, the use of AAS will have caused permanent damage in areas of the brain related to mood and sexual function, which affects 30% of users when AAS are stopped. Their withdrawal is characterized primarily by severe low libido, erectile dysfunction (ED), and depressed mood—symptoms that have been called the "hallmarks" of HPT shutdown. (Kashkin and Kleber,1989; Hochberg et al, 2003; Tan and Scally, 2009; Brower, 2009; Rahnema et al, 2014; Kanayama et al, 2015) When these symptoms are present in a confirmed past or current AAS user, a diagnosis of ASIH can be made with confidence. Regarding the physical exam for hypogonadism, this exam is usually normal if hypogonadism is of recent onset. Diminished facial and body hair, reduced muscle mass, fine facial wrinkles, gynecomastia, and hypotrophic testes are observed in more long-standing and complete ASIH. (Salenave et al, 2012) If observed, these symptoms should be noted and treated. However, the absence of these side effects, which vary with length of AAS use and completeness of testicular shutdown, should neither discourage nor delay an initial diagnosis of

ASIH when acknowledgment of AAS use has been reported and when the hallmark symptoms of ASIH—sexual and mood dysfunction—have been documented. This disease-specific approach to diagnosing ASIH promotes timely medical intervention to relieve suffering and to prevent its potentially harmful sequelae—depression severe enough to prompt use of pain-relieving opioid abuse, or to trigger resumption of AAS use, or even risk suicidality. (Brower, 2009; Kanayama and Brower et al, 2010) Timely, informed diagnosis and treatment provide the optimum chance for reversing damage caused by AAS to the HPT axis. To delay medical intervention by requiring lengthy, expensive, and arguably superfluous diagnostic procedures, which would not change a physician's treatment decision in any event, risks "leaving the body wide open to hormonal collapse" (Turek, 2012) characterized by any- thing from persistent, long-term AAS-induced hypogonadism to permanent testicular shutdown and irreversible (primary) hypogonadism. (Boregowda et al, 2011; Rahnema et al, 2014)   In order to prevent such outcomes, a number of experts have recommended immediate intervention, cautioning that this must not only be timely and symptom focused, but must also continue until symptoms indicate adequate restoration of HPT. (Brower, 2009; Hochberg et al, 2003; Rahnema et al, 2014)

The Role of Labs in Diagnosis and Treatment of ASIH

It is important to recognize that patients who may still be using or have recently used AAS will have testosterone levels that are not valid indicators for clinical decision-making, as these levels will be predictably high. Requiring patients to wait until their current high levels of testosterone fall to hypogonadal levels, per labs, before offering treatment would cause needless suffering, as cessation after years of being on supraphysiological testosterone—whether prescribed or self-administered (i.e., illegal)—predictably results in hypogonadism when these are removed. (Jarow and Lipschultz, 1990; Kanayama et al, 2009; Brower, 2009; Talih et al, 2007; Spratt, 2012; Hochberg et al, 2003) Clearly, requiring patients to go the "cold turkey" route can not only cause unnecessary suffering, but also

89

be physiologically harmful and psychologically dangerous, and it may put patient at risk for re-use, as indicated earlier. A "more rational approach" recommended by a number of experts, is immediate substitution of physiological testosterone to relieve symptoms and support cessation, tapering the dose as HPT function is restored, and/or provision of medications to relieve symptoms, e.g., gynecomastia (tamoxifen), restore fertility (hCG), and encourage restoration of HPT, with the understanding that these medications warrant continuation for as long as they are required. That is, until symptoms indicate adequate restoration of HPT. (Zitzmann and Nieschlag, 2000; Hochberg et al, 2003; Talih et al, 2007; Spratt, 2012; Rahnema et al, 2014)

Of men in the general hypogonadal population who received TRT, 28% began treatment before labs were taken. This may suggest somewhat low confidence by physicians in the diagnostic value of these tests, and more confidence in symptoms. However, while lab values may not be reliable as diagnostic indicators of AAS-related hypogonadism (Wartofsky, 2010), they are important guides for subsequent treatment. For example, after treatment has begun, persistence of symptoms, despite "normal" testosterone levels, could indicate inadequate medications/doses, or severely damaged HPT, and indicate adjustments in the treatment. Finkelstein et al (2013) have reported on the need to asses the role of estrodial as well. Too high lab values during treatment may indicate either use of illegal steroids and ancillary drugs, or too-early lab draws, which can occur when patients do not understand the importance of timely draws.

It's clear that, in addition to understanding hypogonadism, already a complex undertaking, physicians who treat AAS users must also understand this unique form of hypogonadism, ASIH, which, because of its complex pharmacodynamics, presents significant challenges to both diagnosis and treatment.

References

Baggish, A, Weiner, RB, Kanayama, G, Hudson, JI, Lu, MT, Hoffmann, U et al. Cardiovascular toxicity of illicit anabolic-androgenic steroid use, *Circulation,* 2017 May 23;135(21):1991-2002

Barqawi, A, Crawford, ED. Testosterone replacement therapy and the risk of prostate cancer. Is there a link? *Int J Impot Res,* 2006 Jul-Aug;18(4):323-328

Bhasin, S, Pencina, M, Jasuja, GK, Travison, TG, Coviello, A, Orwoll, E et al. Reference ranges for testosterone in men generated using liquid chromatography tandem mass spectrometry in a community-based sample of healthy non-obese young men in the Framingham Heart Study and applied to three geographically distinct cohorts, *J Clin Endocrinol Metab,* 2011 Aug;96(8):2430-2439

Boregowda, K, Joels, L, Stephens, JW, Price, DE. Persistent primary hypogonadism associated with anabolic steroid abuse, *Fertil Steril,* 2011 Jul;96(1):e7-8

Brower, KJ. Anabolic androgenic steroid abuse and dependence in clinical practice, *Phys Sportsmed,* 2009 Dec;37(4):131-140

Canavan, N. Endocrine society pumped up to raise steroid-abuse awareness, *Medscape*, December 17, 2013. http://www.

Caraci, F, Pistarà, V, Corsaro, A, Tomasello, F, Giuffrida, ML, Sortino, MA et al. Neurotoxic properties of the anabolic androgenic steroids nandrolone and methandrostenolone in primary neuronal cultures, *J Neurosci Res,* 2011 Apr; 89(4):592-600

Coward, RM, Rajanahally, S, Kovac, JR, Smith, RP, Pastuszak, AW, Lipshultz, LI. Anabolic steroid induced hypogonadism in young men, *J Urol,* 2013 Dec; 190(6):2200-2205

Crosnoe-Shipley, LE, Elkelany, OO, Rahnema, CD, Kim, ED. Treatment of hypogonadotropic male hypogonadism: case-based scenarios, *World J Nephrol,* 2015 May 6;4(2):245-253

Finkelstein, J, Lee, H, Burnett-Bowie, SA, Pallais, JC, Yu, EW, Borges, LF et al. Gonadal steroids and body composition, strength, and sexual function in men, *N Engl J Med,* 2013 Sep 12;369(11):1011-1022

Gill, GV. Anabolic steroid induced hypogonadism treated with human chorionic gonadotropin, *Postgrad Med J,* 1998 Jan;74(867):45-46

Hochberg, Z, Pacak, K, Chrousos, GP. Endocrine withdrawal syndromes, *Endocr Rev,* 2003 Aug;24(4):523-538

Kanayama, G, Brower, KJ, Wood, RI, Hudson, JI, Pope, HG Jr. Anabolic androgenic steroid dependency: an emerging disorder, *Addiction,* 2009a Dec; 104(12):1966-1978

Kanayama, G, Brower, KJ, Wood, RI, Hudson, JI, Pope, HG Jr. Issues for DSM-V: clarifying the diagnostic criteria for anabolic-androgenic steroid dependence, *Am J Psychiatry,* 2009b Jun;166(6):642-645

Kanayama, G, Brower, KJ, Wood, RI, Hudson, JI, Pope, HG Jr. Treatment of anabolic-androgenic steroid dependence: Emerging evidence and its implications, *Drug Alcohol Depend,* 2010 Jun 1;109(1-3):6-13

Kanayama, G, Hudson, JI, DeLuca, J, Isaacs, S, Baggish, A, Weiner, R, Bhasin, S, Pope, HG Jr. Prolonged hypogonadism in males following withdrawal from anabolic androgenic steroids: an under-recognized problem, *Addiction,* 2015 May;110(5):828-831

Kanayama, G, Hudson, JI, Pope, HG Jr. Long-term psychiatric and medical consequences of anabolic-androgenic steroid abuse: a looming public health concern? *Drug Alcohol Depend,* 2008 Nov 1;98(1-2):1-12

Kanayama, G, Hudson, JI, Pope, HG Jr. Illicit anabolic-androgenic steroid use, *Horm Behav,* 2010 Jun;58(1):111-121

Kashkin, KB, Kleben, HD. Hooked on hormones? An anabolic steroid addiction hypothesis, *JAMA,* 1989 Dec 8;262(22):3166-3170

Kelleher, S et al. Blood testosterone therapy: a European perspective, *J Clin Endocr Metab,* 2004;89(8):3813–3817

Kovac, JR, Scovell, J, Ramasamy, R, Rajanahally, S, Coward, RM, Smith, RP et al. Men regret anabolic steroid use due to a lack of comprehension regarding the consequences on future fertility, *Andrologia,* 2015 Oct;47(8):872-878

Kuhn, C. Anabolic steroids, *Recent Prog Horm Res,* 2002; 7:411-434

Langenbucher, J, Hildebrandt, T, Carr, SJ. Medical consequences of anabolic-androgenic steroid use, in *Handbook of Medical Consequences of Alcohol and Drug Abuse,* J Brick (Ed.). Hawthorne Press: Binghamton, NY, 2004: pp. 325-4

Leone, JE, Sedory, EJ, Gray, KA. Recognition and treatment of muscle dysmorphia and related body image disorders, *J Athl Train,* 2005 Oct-Dec;40(4):352-359

McBride, J, Carson, CC, Coward, RM. Diagnosis and management of testosterone deficiency, *Asian J Androl,* 2015 Mar- Apr;17(2):177-186

McLaren, DS, Brooke, JC, Walter, DJ, Muraleedharan, V, Jones, TH. Long-term effects of testosterone replacement therapy on cardiovascular risk factors in hypogonadism, including men with cardiovascular disease and/or type 2 diabetes, Presented at: *Endocrine Society Annual Meeting,* Houston, TX. June 2012. MON-4

Morgentaler, A 3rd, Conners, WP. Testosterone therapy in men with prostate cancer: literature review, clinical experience, and recommendations, *Asian J Androl,* 2015 Mar-Apr;17(2):206-211

Morgentaler, A. An interview with Abraham Morgentaler, M.D., Harvard Medical School & Public Health. *NEJM,* 2004; 350:48292

Partnership for Drug-Free Kids, 2016

Penatti, CA, Oberlander, JG, Davis, MC, Porter, DM, Henderson, LP. Chronic exposure to anabolic androgenic steroids alters activity and synaptic function in neuroendocrine control regions of the female mouse, *Neuropharmacology,* 2011 Sep;61(4):653-664

Phillips, WN. *Anabolics Reference Guide,* 6th ed. Mile High Publishing; Golden, CO. 1991

Pope, G et al. Adverse health consequences of performance- enhancing drugs: an

Endocrine Society scientific statement, *Endocr Rev,* 2014 Jun;35(3):341-375

Pope, G, Brower, KJ. Treatment of anabolic-androgenic steroid related disorders, Chapter 17, in *The American Psychiatric Publishing Textbook of Substance Abuse Treatment,* eds. M. Galanter, H. Kleber 2008

Rahnema, CD, Crosnoe, LE, Kim, ED. Designer steroids— over-the-counter supplements and their androgenic component: review of an increasing problem, *Andrology,* 2015 Mar;3(2):150-155

Rahnema, C, Lipshultz, LI, Crosnoe, LE, Kovac, JR, Kim, ED. Anabolic steroid induced hypogonadism: diagnosis and treatment, *Fertil Steril.,* 2014 May; 101(5):1271-1279

Salanave, S, Trabado, S, Maione, L, Brailly-Tabard, S, Young, J. Male acquired hypogonadotropic hypogonadism: diagnosis and treatment, *Ann Endocrinol (Paris),* 2012 Apr;73(2): 141-146

Spratt, D. Considering tapering testosterone replacement in certain patients, *Endocr Rev,* September 2012

Talih, F, Fattal, O, Malone, D Jr. Anabolic steroid abuse: psychiatric and physical costs, *Cleve Clin J Med,* 2007 May; 74(5):341-344, 346, 349-352

Tan, RS, Scally, MC. Anabolic steroid-induced hypogonadism— towards a unified hypothesis of anabolic steroid action, *Med Hypotheses,* 2009 Jun;72(6):723-728

Turek, P. Getting off the juice, September 24, 2012. http://www.theturekclinic.com/juice-steroids-anabolics-azoospermia-sterility/

US Department of Justice. Steroid abuse in today's society: a guide for understanding steroids and related substances. March 2004, https://www.deadiversion.usdoj.gov/pubs/brochures/steroids/professionals/

Wartofsky, L, Handelsman, DJ. Standardization of hormonal assays for the 21st century, *J Clin Endocrinol Metab,* 2010 Dec;95(12):5141-5143

WebMD. Deca-durabolin intramuscular side effects. December 17, 2013

WebMD. Dostinex oral, http://www.webmd.com/drugs/2/drug- 14605/dostinex-oral/
details

Wood, RI. Reinforcing aspects of androgens. *Physiol Behav,* 2004 Nov 15;83(2):
279-289

Zitzmann, M, Nieschlag, E. Hormone substitution in male hypogonadism. *Mol Cell
Endocrinol,* 2000 Mar. 30;161(1– 2):73-88

14

AAS Addiction
and Rehab

It's clear that there are serious medical, legal and professional consequences of   AAS. At least for some of their players, professional sports groups can deliver some hefty financial consequences; the armed services take it seriously too—steroids use can result in immediate and dishonorable discharge. Such a weight of consequences suggests appropriate concern about a public health issue; thus, it should be coupled with some serious prevention and intervention efforts, right? To date, however, efforts by these major stakeholders have not been commensurate with the threat contained in growing AAS use across every sector of American life. Still, there are some encouraging signs that this may be beginning to change. For example, the National Institute on Drug Abuse has recently acknowledged the potential for addiction to AAS: "Even though anabolic steroids do not cause the same high as other drugs, steroids are reinforcing and can lead to addiction". (NIDA, 2016) This acknowledgment, and the fact that we now know that at least 3 million Americans are using AAS, with between 15% and 30% likely to become addicted, indicates that the time may have arrived for NIDA and other government health agencies to shift their virtually exclusive focus on AAS use as a law enforcement issue to include significant efforts in prevention and intervention. Such a shift of focus has already begun, along with strong public support,   regarding other prevalent addictions; for example, heroin and opioids.

Several substance abuse experts have supported such a shift, advocating for inclusion of AAS dependency/addiction in the Diagnostic and Statistical Manual of Mental Disorders (DSM). (Kanayama et al, 2009) Research in the fields of endocrinology and neurology has provided insight into unique aspects of AAS addiction which distinguish it from other addictions. For example, while most athletes and clinicians assumed that AAS acted systemically but had little impact on the CNS, a number of studies have now described the neural and endocrinal pathways believed to underlie these unique features of AAS dependency. (Hochberg et al, 2003; Kashkin & Kleber, 1989) It has also been noted that AAS abuse may facilitate the onset or progression of neurodegenerative diseases not usually linked to drug abuse. (Wood, 2004) And it is now recognized that opioids and other similar drugs are often used along with AAS to help with related sleep problems and emotional regulation, thus creating the potential for multi-drug abuse. (NIDA, 2016)

What also distinguishes AAS from other abused substances is the fact that AAS dependency is not characterized by intoxication (highs), but by hypogonadism—the hallmark of AAS use. (Hochberg et al, 2003; Kashkin & Kleber, 1989) And it is this unique form of hypogonadism—anabolic steroid–induced hypogonadism (ASIH)—that plays the major role in AAS addiction. That is, the often overwhelming physiological and psychological symptoms of ASIH are the reasons why users have such difficulty with ending AAS use. Recognizing these unique effects of AAS, and understanding their role in dependency and addiction, is essential to developing protocols for recovery. Unless conventional methods of treating substance abuse are modified for AAS users, they are usually inappropriate. (Brower, 2009)

Sounds like a great challenge for the addiction professionals, doesn't it? Let's take a look at what's available to address this unique addiction. Like any savvy millennial, I began my search with Google: "anabolic steroid recovery." Eureka! Scores of sites to scroll through. However, they all seemed to have the same treatment to offer: month-long stays at often pricey residential treatment centers that had simply tacked "steroid recovery" on to their menu. Reading their prospectus materials made it clear that the menu posting was about as far as most had gone in modifying their operation to meet the needs of AAS addicts. Imagining a patient of mine at one of these places, I didn't know whether to laugh or cry:

> Weighing in at 258 pounds, 33 year old "Johnny" from Chicago has been on AAS for about eight years. He has worked steadily for 15 years at a job he loves, pays his bills, has a loving family, and lives to be big, eat healthy and train hard. As far as he was concerned, he had the best that life could offer, with a raw bench of almost 450 pounds and 20-inch arms. But then something cut that short. Maybe it was his wife or his boss or captain who caught him taking steroids; or maybe his doctor had warned him about a health issue; or maybe he himself had just decided it was time to quit. Johnny had tried to quit a few times already, but withdrawal symptoms made it impossible. He was miserable when his testosterone plummeted to under 100 without the drugs. This time, he decided to seek professional help, and his union was helping with the costs which were not covered by his insurance. Fortunately, he had lots of unused vacation time he could use, so his job was not in jeopardy. As far as his co-workers were concerned, he would be visiting an ailing relative out of town for a month. Going to rehab wasn't something that went down well in Johnny's circle.

> On his first morning at the closest affordable treatment center— 350 miles from his home—Johnny wakes up to a breakfast that included no protein drinks or options for creatine. Okay. He keeps moving through the schedule. It's printed on the cheerful card on his tray. And the staff is just as cheerful, he notes. He hasn't met

the residents yet. Hopefully, they will be cheerful as well. Later that morning, Johnny meets them; in group therapy he openly shares his story. Dr. Bob, the group leader, does his best to find ways for Johnny to find common ground with the cocaine, heroin, and meth lifestyles described by the rest of the group. Johnny thinks they are freaks; they think he is. Though his muscles haven't actually faded much in the two days he's been there without working out, and without steroids or supplements, Johnny thinks he's already getting smaller. The yoga, anti-depressants, and Clomid he was given to help with withdrawal haven't helped; he can't sleep, and he is mirror-checking like never before. Johnny is out of the center long before his month is up. In a few hours, he is back at his gym. Another failed attempt at cessation.

Beyond knowing the dangers of AAS, substance abuse professionals need to know *who their client is* when it comes to AAS addiction. Seeing him or her as another addict, similar to other addicts in self-concept, motivation, and lifestyle, will result in rehabs continuing, with the best of intentions, to offer one-size-fits-all therapy of little use to clients who have become addicted to AAS.

Anyone who has experienced the life of seeking to be the strongest they can be—whose identity *depends* on this— immediately recognizes that rehabs such as I described above have no understanding of who he is and what kind of support he will need as he tries to wean from the drugs that have been part of getting him to look, feel, and be his ideal self. A physician who fully understands AAS and AAS users will also recognize that these professionals do not understand the complexity of the devastating hormonal effects of AAS and why these are the major obstacles to cessation.

Reflecting on the current state of the art in anabolic recovery, I thought especially about the growing numbers of young people who are doing cycle after cycle of AAS, thinking only of the short-term benefits of these drugs. Like most users, teens are unaware that the male hormonal system is so sensitive to AAS that —after even limited AAS use—they may become hypogonadal for a long time, or forever, putting them at risk for dependence or addiction. I thought about how many would one day need rehab as well as specialized medical care for addiction. We need to get our rehab professionals better informed…soon. This is likely to require significant changes in government policies toward AAS.

Harm-Reduction Strategies

"Despite all that is known about the prevalence of AAS use and AAS addiction, the United States' law-and-order approach to reducing the supply of drugs and punishing sellers and users has impeded the development of a public health model to address the crisis". (Neill, 2015) The figures are staggering when one looks at what our government spends on repeated failed versions of the War on Drugs, including attempts to stem steroids use: In 2013, the Obama administration's budget asked for $25.6 billion to fight the drug war, $15 billion of which was directed toward law enforcement. In addition, some $51 billion are spent yearly by state and local governments for drug-related law enforcement. Though it's clear that law enforcement-dominated policies for *all* drugs have failed, there is little sign of introducing meaningful harm reduction into the drug "war." Where such programs do exist, they are generally limited to providing clean needles for intravenous injectors; these programs have been found lacking in capability to provide the wraparound medical, psychological, educational, health, and social services that many addicts need .(Kimergård and McVeigh, 2014) However, even this minimum effort to provide clean needles is not a significant part of government intervention strategy where AAS is concerned. "Although this (harm reduction) approach, more widely accepted in several other countries, has begun to gain some acceptance in the United States, it has not yet made an impact on AAS treatment wherein moral judgments and legal sanctions of drug use (themselves a potential source of harm) have thus far hindered its adoption". (Darkes et al, 2013)

Clearly, there is a disconnect between AAS users and both health providers and

101

government policy. In this vacuum, users continue their reliance on self-help, guided by bro-science which is often itself an obstacle to safe use of AAS, and of virtually no value where addiction is the issue.

References

Brower, KJ. Anabolic androgenic steroid abuse and dependence in clinical practice, *Physician Sports Med*, 2009;37:131-140

Darkes, J et al. Performance-enhancing drug use (including anabolic steroids) by adolescents and college students: etiology and prevention, *Intervention for Addictions*, New York, Academic Press, pp. 833-842, 2013

Hochberg, Z, Pacak, K, Chrousos, GP. Endocrine Withdrawal Syndromes, *Endocr Rev*, 2003 Aug 1;24(4):523–538, https:// doi.org/10.1210/er. 2001-0014

Jarow, JP, Lipshultz, LI. Anabolic steroid-induced hypogonadotropic hypogonadism. *Am J Sports Med*, 1990;18:429

Kanayama, G et al. Issues of DSM-V: Clarifying the diagnostic criteria for anabolic-androgenic dependence, *Am J Psychiatry*, 2009 June 166(6)

Kashkin, KB and Kleber, HD. Hooked on hormones? *JAMA*, 1989 Dec 9;262(22):316-370

Kimergård, A and McVeigh, J. Variability and dilemmas in harm reduction for anabolic steroid users *INHDR Newsletter*, June 2014

Neill, K et al. Tough on drugs: law and order dominance and the neglect of public health in U.S. drug policy, *Journal of World Medical and Health Policy*, September 2015

National Institute on Drug Abuse (NIDA). (2016, March 4). Anabolic Steroids. Retrieved from https://www.drugabuse.gov/publications/ drugfacts/anabolic-steroids on 2017,November 9

Partnership for Drug-Free Kids. Monitoring the Future, *Taylor Hooton Foundation*, 2016

Wood, RI. Reinforcing aspects of androgens, *Physiol Behav,* 2004;83:279-289

15

PCT: Does it Work?

It appears that every AAS user wants to ask about PCT—

regimens for counteracting the hormonal effects of AAS withdrawal at the end of a cycle of use. Online AAS forums are filled with posts about this topic, along with as many differing opinions on how to restore hormonal balance after AAS has depleted endogenous testosterone. In the more than 10 years I've been doing this "Anabolic Doc" thing, I've asked a number of endocrinologists about their take on PCT. Typical response? "PCT? What's that?" So folks, we have a serious issue here. The users who aren't sure about how to do PCT are using all kinds of risky Internet formulas, and the docs who know everything about heart disease, renal failure, diabetes, hypertension, and more esoteric disease states than you can shake a stick at, haven't even heard of PCT. Bill Llewellen, who has been writing about AAS for many years, refers to this in his book, *Anabolics*: "It's amazing how little attention has been paid to hormone normalization in clinical medicine." Actually, I'm more concerned than amazed, given what I've seen as the length of time it can often take organized medicine to recognize and respond to an issue.

The fact that AAS users already number in the millions, with significant numbers who will require medical treatment, including medically supervised PCT, makes a timely response critical.

So, What is PCT?

I have written about this very complex medical issue elsewhere, so I will summarize here:

The sudden cessation of anabolic steroids at the end of a cycle of AAS use, or when a user decides to quit, is associated with a withdrawal phase during which natural testosterone levels remain suppressed for varying amounts of time—some for months, years, or even permanently. As exogenous (artificial) testosterone—AAS—is withdrawn, a patient may experience severe symptoms including fatigue, sexual dysfunction, low mood, depression, and sometimes suicidality. (Canavan, 2013) PCT is used to alleviate these symptoms by helping to restore a man's natural testosterone level, and to mitigate adverse effects of AAS on the body; for example, poor mood and sexual issues, and elevated estrogen levels that can lead to gynecomastia. When to start PCT, what medications to use, and how long to treat is case dependent. Because some PCT medications can disrupt fertility, there are implications for men who wish to remain fertile.

Even this most cursory review of the complexity of the side effects of AAS and attempts to mitigate these should make it clear that managing these effects is not something which can be safely undertaken by anyone without medical training. And yet, every day, AAS users risk their health by taking these drugs and administering their own PCT, informed by the Internet and fellow users, and using products of uncertain ingredients in doses that would terrify anyone familiar with these drugs. Reading the Internet comments of very young users who are doing their own PCT is especially concerning. Even the warnings of older users can't compete with the immortality fantasies of these 18-,

19-, and 20-year old kids who ignore or minimize the future risks of their current behavior.

In my early years of treating men who were using AAS, PCT was a new area of focus for me. These men described their complex self-prescribed PCT regimens which they believed would mitigate the adverse effects of AAS. Often, the very symptoms that brought them to my office contradicted this, and I became determined to learn more about PCT—what men were using, their rationale, and the outcomes. I read everything I could about PCT—I virtually memorized William Llewellyn's *Anabolics*, 9th edition, and I spent countless hours on the Internet reading AAS user blogs. I read whatever journal articles and medical case studies I could find. In addition to this formal and informal data gathering, I picked the brains of patients who were using or had used AAS. Some of these men were pro bodybuilders, powerlifters and strongmen, but—just as is the case today—my typical client was the non- athlete AAS user.

In the medical literature, articles dating back three decades have described the dangerous hormonal side effects of AAS, with many experts also describing medical PCTs which were found to counter withdrawal effects safely and effectively in most cases. Recently, experts have not only validated these earlier findings, but added strong warnings of a burgeoning public health epidemic. These authors, most of whom represent prestigious medical centers, have called for shifts in professional practice and government policy, noting that we have available protocols for safe and effective medically supervised PCT— protocols which have been used successfully both to mitigate the adverse effects of AAS and to support cessation. While there is strong clinical evidence to support these protocols, the lack of any true prospective studies regarding PCT in AAS users has been an obstacle to developing and disseminating evidence-based treatment guidelines for physicians. I am hoping to gain support from the medical community to develop a confidential registry of past and current AAS users as a database with which to do the kind of research that is needed for this. Readers who would be interested in being involved are invited to contact me at tom@toconnormd.com.

Among the medical experts who have encouraged efforts to develop such a registry in order to develop guidelines for medical PCT, and to disseminate these among physicians, is a colleague I greatly admire, Dr. Shalender Bhasin of Harvard Medical School, and Director of the Research Program in Men's Health at Brigham and Women's Hospital. Dr. Bhasin, who was the chairperson of the expert panel convened by the Endocrine Society in 2013 to develop a scientific statement on performance enhancing drugs (PEDs) has a clear grasp of the nature of the AAS epidemic and of the role which physicians—including psychiatrists—must play. In a 2013 interview, he stated:

> "It's not enough to tell someone to stop using anabolic steroids. You can't tell someone to "Just stop doing the drugs." It's not that simple. Sudden cessation of anabolic steroids is associated with a withdrawal phase during which testosterone levels remain suppressed for a varying duration. During this withdrawal phase, the patient may experience severe symptoms of fatigue, sexual dysfunction, low mood, depression and sometimes even suicidality. Some will come through this, even though they will have very distressing symptoms of withdrawal. Some may get into difficulty, and even develop suicidal depression. It's very important to manage the anabolic steroid withdrawal carefully, under the supervision of a team of people, including those who know how to manage body-image disorders.' (Canavan, 2013)

The lack of widely disseminated guidelines and related low levels of AAS awareness among physicians furthers the disconnect between them and users. Therefore, many users will continue to default to risky bro-science to guide them. Ironically, however, this jury-rigged real-world venue could also provide us with in vivo information on what works and what doesn't work, and for which users. Bro-science websites already reveal why men use PCT:

- To restore intact HPTA axis and therefore natural testosterone levels after AAS use
- To mitigate the adverse effects of AAS on the body, such as elevated estrogen levels that can lead to gynecomastia, poor mood, and sexual issues
- To maintain gains in muscle tissue from an AAS cycle

However, because there are no randomized, prospective studies, we do not know if PCT is actually effective in achieving these goals. Based on the numbers of AAS patients I have treated, I can attest to the fact that PCT as we understand it currently does not work for all men. One important reason is that there is so much variability in when, how, and how much AAS was used. In addition to each man's use scenario, his genetics and health history are individual and unique. Many men have come to me and said, "I did my PCT and I'm feeling terrible. What happened, Doc?" I tell them that, as I had explained prior to treatment, I can try to help to relieve their suffering with medically assisted PCT but that there is no guarantee that we will be able to reverse all the damage done to their bodies by AAS. When I see a patient suffering from the side effects of AAS use, I assess his current and past history of AAS use, do a full History and Physical exam, and order and review whatever labs are indicated. Then, we discuss his options—what I call "The Three Doors" of *The Price is Right*.

- Door #1: Stop using AAS.
- Door #2: Wean with medical-grade PCT.
- Door #3: Wean with androgens.

These "doors" cover any man suffering from the side effects of AAS use.

Weaning with Medically Supported PCT

A popular PCT regimen includes selective estrogen receptor modulators (SERMs), human chorionic gonadotropin (HCG), and anti-estrogen medications called aromatase inhibitors (AIs). But what is the *best* PCT regimen? Again, there is no consensus on this, but I believe that William Llewellyn has the best answer: "After an AAS cycle that is 'suppressive', the testes will definitely need pharmacologic stimulation with supraphysiologic doses of luteinizing hormone LH analog-HCG for some time." How long? What dose? And when should the dosing start after an AAS cycle? All of this will depend on personal aspects of the individual AAS user, but I agree that medically supported PCT should start after the AAS testosterone ester is about at its 25% half-life to ensure that the overlap is adequate to reduce suffering. I also believe that dosing should take place for about 2 weeks, and that the most important medications will be the SERMs family.

I do not agree with the use of AIs for medically supported PCT. After hearing of many men experiencing heart attacks that I believe were secondary to AI use, I do not routinely use AIs. In certain clinical situations, however, very light AI use can relieve suffering.

Currently, many experts recommend using only one SERM and not, as Llewellen recommends, using clomiphene and tamoxifen at the same time. I agree with Llewellyn. Having seen seeing hundreds of men on his regimen (or a similar one), I have found that these end results are best. The combination regimen optimizes the re-start of the HPTA axis and eases the desensitization effects of what the HCG has done to the LH receptor in the testes. I recommend concluding the end of medical PCT cycle with tamoxifen, as I have found that the anti-estrogenic effects of extended use of clomiphene on the hypothalamus/

pituitary by AAS users versus non-users (hypogonadal men without prior AAS use) will lead to sexual dysfunction. This clinical discovery has led me to favor limiting or even eliminating clomiphene from medical monitored PCT cycles. I have also developed some of my own regimen/doses for patients who are on fixed doses of testosterone for life. Interesting and novel, these are related to long-term suppression of the HPTA axis, testicular atrophy, and cholesterol synthesis. Let me emphasize, however: *Each medical PCT regimen has to be personalized for each man.* I also continue to say that, at the end of the day, you will have to take off the training wheels (PCT) to see if your intact HPTA axis has what it takes to produce adequate androgen.

References

Canavan, N. Endocrine society pumped up to raise steroid-abuse awareness. Medscape, Dec.17, 2013. http://www.medscape.com/viewarticle/817960

Kanayama, G et al. Treatment of AAS dependency: emerging evidence and its implications, *Drug Alcohol Depend,* 2010 Jun1;109(13):6-13

Llewellyn, W. *Anabolics*, 9th ed. Jupiter, FL: Molecular Nutri- tion; 2009

16

Tales
From the
Underground

Here is a reflection on an entry in my journal from a few years back. I think it reflects the spiritual context for my professional and personal interest in what I call "Big Medicine"—the care of the strength athlete.

"Got restless in the clinic, and I thought it was time to see some of my lifter patients in their own environments. So I planned a road trip, taking my buddy Adam along. Adam, the kid who benches 600 pounds, and I took off at 5:30 a.m. in my "Mac-Daddy" Suburban. Drove north for about four hours. Drank untold numbers of cups of coffee, multiple grams of creatine products, NO vasodilators, more BCAAs than my muscles could absorb, and Adam had us breathing Nose-Tork at every toll!

We were out to train with one of the most hardcore hellbent powerlifters

113

on the planet—Bill Crawford, who is a world-class bench presser. We pull up to this old-school gym. It's always "old school" but God, it gives me butterflies in my stomach every time I walk into these places. Ever since I was a kid, walking up those stairs to the gym, smelling the Ben-Gay and hearing those plates banging, my limbic brain tunes up, and I'm ready to rock…We walk in…"What's up!" "Hey Doc, you're late, get changed and let's go!" We enter the weight room, and a couple of the guys meet us—damn, I've seen these guys in *Powerlifting USA* – cool! We focus on two large custom bench presses, an unloaded bar, and a lot of 100-pound plates. I don't know about my buddy Adam, but I'm nervous. You don't really know where to stand or where to put your gear. Then some big man tells us to stand back as he shuffles through CDs overhead, like some muscle-bound Grand Master Flash, as he creates the music selection for the training day. BOOOOM— for the next two hours, we train with music so loud that we're lip reading each other. I loved it—totally old-school! The WHO, Black Sabbath, Led Zeppelin, Nirvana, Hendrix, Slip Knot, Static-X, and even some of that funky Metal/Rap stuff. Bottom line, my motor end plates were fired up big time while I benched up to 405 x reps off the boards. (I was the weakest guy in the gym – thank God, I have a big ego.) Adam turned a few heads with his raw 475 pounds to the chest. And we watched firsthand the big men benching up to 850 to the chest. What an experience. Religious. We did our thing and completed the training day with some real cool "West Side" regimens and then someone finally turned the music down and said hello to us."

So, there it is! For those who don't understand us and why we do what we do, imagine the hardcore opera singer or fan who belts out their song with as much effort as a big bencher. That's right, what's the difference? Same passion, same dedication... same thrill. Not the same risks, though. And that reminds me to put on my lab coat and get into some real "hardcore" medicine that may save your life.

17

Becoming the Metabolic Doc

P owerlifters are the poster boys and girls for the proverbial "Never say die."
"Never enough; go bigger, stronger" is the mantra. This is not a sport for the
faint of heart—or light of limb. Powerlifting is an "extreme" sport with its own
extreme culture. The very name reveal the goal: Lift heavy; lift heavier; then
lifter even heavier. While there are obvious medical/physiological consequences
of "lifting big," these receive scant attention in the medical community apart
from orthopedic surgeons (who know all about re-inserting ruptured biceps
tendons). But, as any lifter knows, this isn't the only item on the list of medical
problems that strongmen encounter. Problems that affect the heart, blood vessels,
kidneys, and liver are endemic to heavy lifting and its attendant lifestyle. These
are the purview of internal medicine; yet this very critical medical specialty is
largely missing in action where the powerlifting population is concerned.

Let me give you the short version of how I became the Metabolic Doc: As
both a heavy lifter and an internal medicine physician, I have a special interest in
the metabolic health of fellow lifters—a group that is known to have shortened
life spans secondary to untreated hypertension, enlarged hearts, and the

metabolic derangements seen all too frequently in "big" people. By adapting medical protocols to the needs of lifters, I have been able to successfully manage these problems without causing weakness—the bane of the lifter's life.

18

Blood Clots and the "Mass Effect" In Big Men

The term *blood clot* refers to a condition in which blood clumps together and causes a blockage somewhere in the body's blood vessels. The medical term for this condition is *hypercoagulability,* and it can occur in either the arteries or the veins. When clots form in the veins, it is known as deep venous thrombosis (DVT). You may have heard of this occurring to a passenger during or after a lengthy plane ride. The risk of DVT is that the clot will travel to the lungs and cause a pulmonary embolism (PE), a potentially fatal medical condition that is seen in hospitalized patients who spend a great deal of time in bed. Reports of fatalities in heavy lifters always bring this to mind for me. This may have been what happened to some of the powerlifters who suffered early deaths. Without their physicians' statements, I can't say for sure, but the report of a blood clot makes me think "pulmonary embolism." Blood clots are something I am ever watchful for in my patients who use AAS. Among this group, it is more common to think of an arterial (as opposed to venous) clot, which causes a blockage called a thrombosis and which can lead to a heart attack or stroke.

There are several characteristics common to arterial and venous clots. Though the mechanism(s) of DVT/PE and arterial thrombosis have been well studied, their relationship to AAS use specifically has not been examined. I decided to write this chapter because I believe that most physicians are not aware of the relationship of blood clots to AAS use. So, it wasn't surprising that I was not able to find a single study that discussed the relationship of AAS and hypercoagulability. My discussion on this topic will therefore be based on what is known about DVT and PE generally and what I have observed in my clinical practice with lifters.

The hypercoagulable state is reached through different means when it affects the arteries or veins, but we know that on the arterial side, the basic components of the metabolic syndrome—that is, a combination of high blood pressure (hypertension), diabetes, and lipid abnormalities—plays the main role. In addition to metabolic syndrome, AAS users encounter several other medical problems:

- Polycythemia (heavy blood)
- Decreased HDL and increased LDL cholesterol
- Elevated and labile hypertension causing adverse sheering forces on the endothelial lining
- Increases in pro-inflammatory cytokines (blood products produced in the liver and the endothelial lining of the blood vessels), including an increase in hypercoagulable factors and a reduction of natural anticoagulants
- Increased oxidative stress to the endothelial

lining.

- Adverse renal function, including nephrotic syndrome and loss of protective blood proteins (see chapter on anabolic cardio-renal syndrome)
- Elevated estrogen (when on AAS, one's estrogen levels are proportionally elevated in a dose-dependent fashion, which has been shown in studies of women on hormone replacement therapy to cause blood clots)

In men, AAS abolishes follicle-stimulating hormone (FSH) and luteinizing hormone (LH), potentially resulting in the creation of clots. Studies have demonstrated that AAS can lead to direct adverse effects on the endothelial lining and myocardial tissue—what I call the "mass effect" on the body— meaning that when you are "big" and on AAS, the hemodynamic physics gets worse. For example, left ventricular hypertrophy is a classic known risk for heart attack and stroke—and let's not forget to mention obstructive sleep apnea (OSA). Did you know that AAS can cause and worsen OSA? The takeaway of all of this is, first and foremost, **DON'T USE AAS IF YOU DON'T WANT TO TAKE THESE RISKS!**

If you do decide to use AAS, beware. Other important recommendations include seeing a doctor, and being honest with him or her so they can get a good history and physical exam done. Be sure to include any family history of hypercoagulability. There are well-known, common genes and familial conditions that cause clotting (factor V Leiden is the most common, numbering about 3 million cases annually). Prothrombin gene mutation, deficiencies in protein S, protein C, anti-thrombin, and dysfibrinogenemia are others. If you are not sure your doctor is familiar with all of this, see a hematologist or cardiologist.

What Can You Do to Reduce These AAS-Associated Risks?

Those of you who are familiar with my work know that I hammer on staying as healthy as you can during your quest for strength and size. So, once again, I am writing about the relationship of AAS and blood clots. Many well-trained doctors are not aware that blood clots are one of the many serious side effects of AAS. If it were not for my own life-log fascination with strength sports and respect for those who participate in them—and yes, my special interest in Men's Health—I too might be unaware. And here again, I will repeat what I have so often said, First, keep your doses down, treat hypertension, and address your poor lipid profiles. My experience has demonstrated that an AAS-knowledgeable physician and good follow-up can get almost anyone to goal!

Next, check your labs for polycythemia, liver and renal function, lipids, and low vitamin D. (Vitamin D has been shown to have an anticoagulant effect.) Talk with your doctor about using low-dose aspirin, which acts as a blood thinner and can help reduce the risk of blood clots. Note that this recommendation is controversial now as it is not such a simple matter. Ditto for the decision to have red wine every day; you have probably heard wine has some good health benefits, but it also has some drawbacks. Finally, talk with your doctor about treating low vitamin D. Ask if you should try coenzyme 10 and fish oil, and if you can safely increase your cardio.

19

HGG, Heart Health and Bodybuilders: Strange Bedfellows

Human growth hormone (HGH) and variant sub-types of insulin- like growth factor-1 (IGF-1) have been used in bodybuilding and athletics as well as in anti-aging clinics, around the world for over 20 years. Virtually every gym rat knows someone who is on HGH or an IGF-1 subtype. The most popular of these is IGF-1 Lr3, which is essentially more powerful IGF-1. This variant has been chemically altered to be more potent and has an in- creased half-life from 12 to 20 hours (vs. 20 minutes for standard IGF-1), making the effects of this agent outlast and outperform straight HGH or IGF-1. There are many anecdotal reports of men spot-injecting this form of IGF-1 and seeing their arms swell up to 2 inches while working out.

IGF-1 Lr3 appears to bind better than IGF-1 to cellular IGF- 1R receptors in skeletal muscle, leading to increases in protein synthesis and an enhanced transcription factor that helps to regulate the expression of genes. This kind of result, with and without other AAS, is the holy grail for bodybuilders.

With results like this, it would seem like this stuff really works. But, because of all the other AAS being used by these individuals, it's hard to know which one (or which combination) is really producing an effect. Or is it the hard training? The steroid stacks? Or perhaps the insulin, pro-hormones, food, protein, and pre/post supplements? Is HGH/IGF-1 actually helping to grow all the muscle we see in these huge guys? With so many possible confounders, it's impossible to know.

The medical literature provides ample evidence that HGH is indeed anabolic and leads to improvements in metabolic synergy—that is, added muscle and reduction of fat in the abdomen. But to what extent does this occur? In whom? And what are the side effects? These questions remain unanswered, and the kind of human studies required to provide these answers would be unethical. We are left with mostly anecdotal evidence that HGH and IGF-1 work.

One does have to wonder why, in spite of the fact that these agents are known to be so widely used, there has been so little medical curiosity about their muscle-building properties. We know more about the fruit fly's genome than we do about if and how HGH works to build muscle. If there is any validity to the anecdotal reports of muscle growth, think about its potential as a treatment for any number of muscle-wasting diseases.

Although the muscle-building effects of HGH and the IGF-1 agents are not being widely explored, there is keen interest in the effects of these agents on other medical conditions, for example, heart disease. A number of studies report that GH/IGF-1 axis regulates cardiac growth, stimulates heart muscle contractility, and influences the vascular system. (Andreassen et al, 2009; Castellano et al, 2009; Troncoso et al, 2014; Ungvari and Csiszar 2012) Chronic GH excess has also been associated with acromegaly, a condition that affects the heart and produces morphological abnormalities; that is, abnormalities in cardiac muscle structure and function, inducing a specific cardiomyopathy. GH excess appears to actually enhance cardiac performance in early-stage acromegaly, but as the condition advances the cardiac effects become adverse, potentially progressing to heart failure. In a 2010 report, Meinhardt and colleagues provide this description of GH deficiency:

"Growth hormone deficiency (GHD) produces different clinical features depending on the time of onset and disease severity and duration. GHD negatively affects cardiovascular function by directly acting on the heart and endothelium (blood vessels); it also acts indirectly by causing insulin resistance, abdominal obesity, hypercoagulability, increase in serum lipids, reduction in exercise performance, and pulmonary capacity. GHD patients have increased total body fat, atherothrombotic and proinflammatory abnormalities, dyslipidemia, and decreased insulin-stimulated glucose uptake by fat and skeletal muscle. In addition to the cardiovascular risk factors mentioned above, GHD patients have increased vessel intima-media thickness, which is the earliest morphological change in the development of atherosclerosis—clinical heart disease."

Atherosclerosis, a condition in which plaque builds up inside the arteries, can lead to heart attacks, strokes, or even death. Researchers at the University of Missouri (Ungvari and Csiszar, 2012) have found that IGF-1, a protein which is found naturally in high levels in adolescents, can help prevent arteries from clogging. Other researchers found that increasing atherosclerosis patients' levels of the protein could reduce the amount of plaque buildup in their arteries, lowering their risk of heart disease. "The body already works to remove plaque from arteries through certain types of white blood cells called macrophages," said Yusuke Higashi, PhD, assistant research professor in the Division of Cardiovascular Medicine at the Mississippi University School of Medicine. "However, as we age, macrophages are not able to remove plaque from the arteries as easily. Our findings suggest that increasing IGF-1 in macrophages could be the basis for new approaches to reduce clogged arteries

123

and promote plaque stability in aging populations."

Because it appears that as we grow older we lose levels of IGF-1, safely increasing these levels and maintaining a sustained physiologic balance might provide protection against heart disease and other age-related conditions. Because IGF-1 analogs like IGF-1 Lr3 are inexpensive and readily available, this possibility is intriguing. Questions that need to be answered include: Is it simply that we can use HGH and or IGF-1 analogs like IGF-1 Lr3 to increase or supplant natural levels of IGF-1? What are the correct regimens? What are the side effects of such therapies? What role would this play in delivering ethical medical care to everyone in our society?

One thing I can tell you is that nothing in the medical world is a simple slam-dunk. It will most likely end up that there are certain people, at certain critical times, receiving specified regimens of HGH/IGF-1 analogs like IGF-1 Lr3 that will benefit from the research and clinical applications that we could be working on now. These would build on the many studies demonstrating that regulating a balance between IGF-1 levels is the key to using HGH and/or IGF-1 analogs to protect against heart disease and, perhaps even more significantly, that patients with heart disease—specifically those in heart failure—have responded favorably to HGH therapy.

References

Andreassen, M et al. IGF-1 as predictor of all cause mortality and cardiovascular disease in an elderly population, *Eur J Endocrinol,* 2009 Jan;160(1):25-31

Castellano, G, Affuso, F, Conza, PD, Fazio, S. The GH/IGF-1 axis and heart failure. *Curr Cardiol Rev,* 2009 Aug;5(3):203- 215

Meinhardt, U et al. The effects of growth hormone on body composition and physical performance in recreational athletes:a randomized trial, *Ann Intern Med,* 2010 May4;152(9): 568-577

Ungvari, A and Csiszar, A. The emerging role of IGF-1 deficiency in cardiovascular aging: recent advances, *J Gerontol A Biol Sci Med Sci,* 2012 Jun;67(6):

599-610

Troncoso, R, Ibarra, C, Vicencio, JM, Jaimovich, E, Lavandero, S. New insights into IGF-1 signaling in the heart. *Trends Endocrinol Metab,* 2014 Mar; 25(3):128-137

20

Anabolic Cardiorenal Syndrome

Some of you may remember an Anabolic Doc article in which I presented an anonymized clinical case called, "Lifer's Endothelial Cardiomyopathy", a unique version of cardiorenal syndrome which is commonly seen in AAS users. My experience with large numbers of AAS and lifter patients helped me to develop the case management protocol I employed in this case—including a system of data collection which elicits the range of information needed to diagnose and treat this typically multi-factorial disease which is found in lifters—both AAS using and non-using. As background, I will present some short excerpts from the medical literature which describe cardiorenal syndrome as a bi-directional model that leads to the demise of both the heart and kidney simultaneously. (Bongartz et al, 2005)

Stevenson and colleagues explain the importance of understanding the bi-directionality of cardiorenal syndrome:

> *"The view of the kidney as a simple filter suffering the ill effects of a failing pump has been challenged as our understanding of the complex interactions between these organs grows. Both organs are regulators of vital functions*

127

—for example, blood pressure, vascular tone, diuresis, natriuresis, circulating volume homeostasis, peripheral perfusion and tissue oxygenation. Both have endocrine functions and are capable of cellular and humoral signaling. The interplay of these organs is clear in many instances and dysfunction of the other." (Stevenson et al, 2005)

Kimmenade and colleagues describe the interplay:

"Changes in the function of one organ can lead to a spiral of dysfunction in both, through altered balance between nitric oxide and reactive oxygen species, systemic inflammation, [and] activation of both the sympathetic nervous system and the renin-angiotensin- aldosterone system (RAAS). We now know that in the setting of kidney dysfunction, the heart experiences varying degrees of accelerated atherosclerosis, left ventricular hypertrophy and remodeling, myocardial micro-angiopathy, and vascular calcification—while in the setting of cardiac dysfunction, hypoperfusion and excessive activation of the RAAS contribute to contribute to progressive renal insufficiency." (Kimmenade et al, 2006)

Bongartz and colleagues describe those at highest risk for this disease: *"Individuals with the constellation of potentially modifiable risk factors for cardiovascular disease are also at higher risk for renal disease, as many of these factors such as smoking, hypertension, dyslipidaemia, age, ANABOLIC STEROID USE (my emphasis), and diabetes are also factors in the progression of renal disease".* (Bongartz et al, 2005)

Case Study

AB, a 40-year-old Caucasian male, presents with 10 years of AAS use and progressive malaise and fatigue.

History of Present Illness:

Over the past year, AB has found himself getting more tired, with a noted decline in his ability to perform in the gym and in daily activities. He notes daily headaches, occasional dizziness, increased shortness of breath, and general weakness. He denies chest pain, nausea, and abdominal pain, but he does complain of pain in his back, knees, and left shoulder.

Past Medical History:

One episode of acute renal failure; general arthritis in his cervical spine, with neck pain and low back pain; hypertension; elevated cholesterol; obstructive sleep apnea; ruptured distal biceps tendon, right side status post-repair. Denies any hospitalizations/blood transfusions, and has a spleen.

Psycho-Social History:

AB is married and has three children. Works as an office manager. Denies any environmental exposure and does not smoke or abuse alcohol/drugs, although he tells me that he has used cocaine in the remote past. He has been using AAS for about 10 years, with almost no time off. His AAS use has been testosterone, mixed blends and Cypionate, about 300 mg q 6 days intramuscular injection (IM). He also adds Deca-Durabolin, about 300-400 mg IM q week. He has used various oral AAS, HGH and PCT with HCG and Clomid over the years. His weight training is intense and strong. He does not do any cardiovascular training at all. I noted that AB is a "very type A" male; in my office he was hyper-alert and not relaxed.

Family Medical History:

AB tells me that both of his parents have issues with elevated cholesterol and blood pressure. There is coronary artery disease and hypertension in some first degree relatives.

Medications:

AB is not currently on any meds, although he was prescribed "something for his blood pressure" several years ago. He takes a multivitamin, creatine, and protein powder before, and at times after workouts; and uses AAS, as above. Denies any known drug allergies.

Review of Systems:

On review of body systems, AB mentions that he has had very poor sleep over the past year or so, with periods of what appears to be apnea. He is very tired during the day; short of breath with light activity; complains of heartburn at night; has occasional swelling of his lower limbs; dizzy spells in the gym after heavy sets; and urinates several times per night. He also complains of erectile issues.

Physical Exam:

Vitals signs showed a heart rate of 90 beats per minute and blood pressure of 150/110. A very muscular man in no apparent distress, AB is 5'9" and weighs 236 pounds. His neck size is 18" and abdomen is 44".

Cardiovascular exam revealed no murmurs; lungs were clear on auscultation; gynecomastia and nipple tenderness were noted. No abnormalities of the abdomen, including palpation of liver and spleen. His testes were atrophied on exam and his prostate was slightly enlarged on digital rectal exam. He had trace edema of his bilateral ankles. His neurologic exam was within normal limits.

Lab & Diagnostic Studies:

Cholesterol panel shows a total of 287, HDL of 9, triglycerides of 198, and an LDL of 238; CHO/HDL ratio of 31.9. On CBC, hematocrit was 52%; comprehensive metabolic panel shows an elevated creatinine of 1.7, AST of 65; urinalysis shows trace protein. Vitamin D, low at 13 ng/mL. ECG shows a normal sinus rhythm with possible signs of LVH (enlarged heart).

Echocardiogram shows enlargement of LV with mildly reduced systolic function.

Stress test showed findings suggestive of non-ischemic cardio-myopathy. Sleep study shows moderate obstructive sleep apnea.

Diagnosis/Analysis and Plan:

AB has a form of cardiorenal syndrome I call "Lifter's Endothelial-Cardiomyopathy"—heart disease secondary to a combination of long-term uncontrolled hypertension, abnormalities in lipids, and obstructive sleep apnea, with AAS having played a role in the pathophysiology. This case illuminates the multi-factorial nature of cardiorenal syndrome as it occurs in lifters who use AAS (and some who don't). Treatment, which was successful, required addressing several medical issues, coordinating with other physicians where needed, and significant changes regarding AB's use of AAS. Patient, who has now been on stable, medically monitored and managed doses of HRT for three years, continues to lift and to be strong. His cardiologist reported recently that AB's echocardiogram indicated that his heart was now normal.

This patient was fortunate to have received timely medical attention from a physician who was well informed on diagnosis and treatment of the complex effects of heavy lifting as well as AAS use.

In summary, AAS can cause medical conditions that will hurt the heart and kidneys through hypertension, abnormalities in lipid physiology, accelerated oxidation, and vascular inflammation, not to mention a laundry list of direct biologic cytokines (signaling molecules) that will wreak havoc on your heart and kidney.

How to minimize these interactions?

- **Do NOT use AAS.** After years of using AAS and supra- physiologic doses of hormone replacement therapy, some men manifest some type of metabolic disease— including heart failure (both diastolic and systolic), heart attacks, strokes, peripheral vascular disease, erectile dysfunction, and acute/chronic kidney disease.

- **If you use AAS, keep your doses down, limit the time you use, and above all, stay heart healthy**. Make sure your blood pressure and lipid panel are optimal by eating a healthy diet, doing cardiovascular exercise, and (as needed) taking medications prescribed by a doctor who is aware of your risk factors and keeps you informed.

You can be big and strong without sacrificing your health to your goal!

References

Bongartz, LG, Cramer, MJ, Doevendans, PA, Joles, JA, The severe cardiorenal syndrome: Guyton revisited, *Eur Heart J,* 2005 Jan; 26(1): 11-17

Kimmenade, RR, Januzzi, JL Jr, Baggish, AL, Lainchbury, JG, Bayes-Genis, A, Richards, AM. Amino-terminal pro-brain natriuretic peptide, renal function, and outcomes in acute heart failure: redefining the cardiorenal interaction? *J Am Coll Cardiol,* 2006 Oct 17;48(8):1621-1627

Stevenson, LW, Nohria, A, Mielniczuk, L. Torrent or torment from the tubules? Challenge of the cardiorenal connections. *J Am Coll Cardiol,* 2005 Jun 21;45(12):2004-2007

21

Hardcore Medicine: The Case of Heavy-Duty Blood and the Lifter

Let's look at another interesting, esoteric but common medical problem I see regularly in men who use AAS—"heavy duty blood" which is known as polycythemia secondary to AAS use.

Chief Complaint

JD, a 34-year-old Caucasian male, was found to have an abnormal complete blood count (CBC) when he saw his previous doctor.

History of Current Illness

Over the last 4 months, JD has had frequent headaches, blurred vision, and general malaise. He has been using AAS for 10 years. JD just completed a very long cycle consisting of several intramuscular (IM) and oral AAS. After winning an important bodybuilding show, he decided to see his doctor for his current symptoms. His doctor completed general lab work and found some tests to be abnormal; the most significant was a hematocrit of 57.2%. At this point, JD made an appointment to see me. He wanted to know if his symptoms were related to his AAS use. He had not told his doctor about his use, and the doctor did not ask.

Review of Systems

In addition to the headaches that have been waking him up at night, JD complained of night sweats, progressive malaise, and general weakness in the gym. He denied chest pain, palpitations, or nausea, but did mention that he has lost weight—about 20 pounds—over the past 2 months. He also complained of poor libido and erection issues.

Past Medical/Surgical History

Significant for untreated hypertension and an abnormal cholesterol panel, with a very elevated LDL and a very low HDL, gastroesophageal reflux disease (GERD), abnormal levels of liver enzymes (Gilbert's syndrome), exercise-induced asthma, right shoulder arthroscopic surgery for rotator cuff injury, and chronic low back pain. He sustained a right quad rupture in the past.

Medications (including AAS, Supplements, and Past Medications)

At the time I took JD's history, he was on testosterone cypionate 400 mg intramuscular (IM) injection once a week and Deca-Durabolin 300 mg (IM) every 5 days. He has been on this dose for about 2 months. In the past 2 years, he has been as much as much as 1,800 mg of testosterone per week and has used multiple types of AAS including Dianabol, Anadrol-50, Finaplix, Masteron, Equipoise, insulin, and HGH. He ran PCT with Arimidex, HCG, and Clomid. All these drugs were obtained from underground sources. He was on no medications from his doctors.

Drug Allergies

Sulfa meds

Psychosocial History

He works in IT. He does not smoke and reports occasional alcohol use.
He does not use recreational drugs and has no environmental exposures.

Family Medical History

JD's mother and father are in relatively good health, with some hypertension and high cholesterol (hypercholesterolemia). He states that he thinks that a relative with a blood disorder.

Laboratory Studies, Tests, and Clinical Procedures

CBC indicates clear polycythemia with an HCT of 57.2% and a hemoglobin of 19.4 g/d; normal mean corpuscular volume (MCV)

- Creatinine of 1.5, and an estimated glomerular filtration rate (an indicator of kidney health) of 50 mL/ min/1.73 m^2
- Liver function tests are elevated with an aspartate aminotransferase (AST) value of 150 units per liter
- Total testosterone over 3,000 ng/dL and total estrogen over 300 pg/mL
- Urinalysis shows 1+ protein
- Heterozygous for the *H63D* mutation in the *HFE* gene
- Electrocardiograph shows sinus rhythm with evidence of left ventricular hypertrophy (enlarged heart)
- Echocardiogram shows enlarged left ventricle and diastolic dysfunction

Vital Signs
- Height 5'11"/Weight 215 pounds

- Blood pressure 150/110
- Waist 41"

Physical Exam
Within normal limits

Analysis of Case

JD, whose case details were similar to many men who use AAS, was found to be sensitive to androgens with regard to their potential for causing overproduction of red blood cells (erythrocytosis/ polycythemia), a potentially fatal condition related to hereditary hemochromatosis (HH). HH is a disorder that causes the body to absorb too much iron from the diet. It is one of the most common genetic disorders in the United States, affecting about 1 million people. It most often affects people of Northern European descent. Research has found that Caucasians present with much higher red blood cell tests than other racial groups (Acton et al, 2006). I have seen this difference in AAS patients across several racial groups.

With HH, the excess iron is stored in the body's tissues and organs, particularly the skin, heart, liver, pancreas, and joints. Because humans cannot increase the excretion of iron, excess iron can overload and eventually damage tissues and organs. For this reason, HH is also called an iron overload disorder. In addition to causing heart disease, liver disease, and testicular failure, men with elevated HCTs are at risk for strokes. JD, however, does not have HH but, as stated, is sensitive to the polycythemia effects of AAS use.

The takeaway of this case is this: if you are on AAS, please have your doctor run a CBC. If, like JD, you may have the genetic potential to be sensitive to AAS, certain types of AAS can really harm you. The fact that Caucasians typically present with much higher red blood cells doesn't mean that AAS users from other racial or ethnic groups may not also develop this disorder.

I recommend that all users have their CBC checked during the max point of a cycle. And, PLEASE, be wary of the gym gurus who may try to help you understand your labs!

References

Acton, RT et al. Geographic and racial differences in HFE mutation in the hemochromatosis and iron overload screening (HEIRS) study, *Ethnic Dis*, 2006 Autumn;16(4):815-821

22

Hypertension in the Powerlifter: Diagnosis and Treatment

Hypertension is one of the most common dangerous medical conditions affecting powerlifters. When lifters are young (35 or under), and lean, hypertension is rare, but as the lifter gets older, and larger, he (and yes, she) can become hypertensive. At least 75% of my male lifter patients over age 40 who train at body weights over 220 pounds are hypertensive, with blood pressures (BPs) over 130/80, per the latest guidelines published by NIH in November 2017. This is stage 1 hypertension. Mind you, this is their resting BP, not what the lifter's BP is during training, which is obviously much higher. (note: in November, 2017, NIH issued new guidelines for defining hypertension: 130/80 mm Hg, rather than 140/90 mm Hg)

Living with hypertension long enough can lead to premature heart disease and stroke, and it commonly causes an enlarged heart (called left ventricular hypertrophy or LVH), which is a very dangerous condition leading to congestive heart failure and death. Please note that in this chapter, I discuss LVH that occurs as a result of hypertension and not as a result of heavy lifting or strenuous exercise. Here, I am discussing pathologic LVH secondary to hypertension.

The mechanisms underlying the development of hypertension-related LVH are multifactorial and have not been fully elucidated. But one thing you can be sure of is that if you are a lifter with hypertension, your days of smashing weights will be limited compared to a lifter with a normal BP—the normotensive lifter.

So, what is a hypertensive lifter to do? Here is your checklist:

See your doctor and have your BP checked.

If your arms are 17 inches or more, make sure your BP is monitored with a large adult cuff. Small cuffs can lead to falsely elevated levels. Sometimes, we doctors see "white-coat hypertension" in the clinic (presumably as a result of the stress of being in a doctor's office), which is not representative of the patient's usual BP. You might want to buy a good home monitor or, better yet, ask an RN friend to check your BP. I ask my patients to check their BPs at home first thing in the morning, again some time in the late afternoon, and then again at bedtime.

Take the average of these three readings, and be sure to check BOTH arms. If there is more than a 15% difference in the readings between your arms, see a doctor right away. You may have a medical condition that needs further investigation.

Limit your salt intake to less than 1,500 mg per day.

We have known for many years that salt contributes to hypertension. The Mediterranean Diet can cure hyper- tension and is without doubt the best diet to protect any- one's heart. I live by this diet and frequently recommend that patients try to follow it as well.

Exercise Regularly

The dual cornerstones of heart health are diet and exercise. However, powerlifting is not exactly the gold standard for cardio protective exercise. I say that as a powerlifter myself, one who has been smashing weights for over 35 years and who now, at age 52, is still getting stronger. So I understand the desire to lift BIG, but as a physician I also understand that lifting big weights for years can lead to hypertension, and untreated hypertension can lead to heart disease.

What's the best way to tailor your powerlifting routine to avoid hypertension and heart disease? Try to *train at the lightest body weight you can.* Some of my power lifting patients laugh when I ask them to wean down to lower and lower weight classes (you guys know who you are!). I've had guys go from 308 pounds to 242, and even as low as 220—and actually get stronger!Next, go for high intensity interval training (HIIT). Pay attention here—this is important. None of us lifters are going to go out and run a couple of miles before a big bench or squat day. Actually, I'm very much against running or lifting after cardio. Remember, I come from the old school and the days when no one dreamed of doing cardio at a power lifting gym. These days I get my cardio on a mountain bike in the woods. That's about as sophisticated as I get with my HIIT. If all you do-- with your physician's approval-- is some form of cardio at least four times a week, at a modest intensity for 25 minutes, it should be enough to keep your BP down.

A reminder: I write to educate, not to treat. My articles—and this book —are in no way meant to substitute for the advice of your personal doctor.

Lest the point be missed: SEE YOUR DOCTOR for advice about *your* particular situation. Share with him or her what you read here as you discuss your symptoms and numbers. If you and your doctor find that your BP will not come down, discuss the possible need for a BP medication.

As a physician specifically trained in managing hypertension, I can state with confidence that it is incredibly important to choose BP medicine that is specific to an individual's physiology and needs. One size most certainly does NOT fit all. There are four BP drugs that I use I use in about 98% of my hypertensive lifters. Two are HCTZ and amlodipine. The other two, and the ones I use most commonly, are ACE inhibitors and a very special cardio-selective nitric oxide-donating agent called Bystolic. I've had great success with these agents. Another interesting fact about Bystolic is that it can act like a weak Viagra! This effect has been well known for years in Europe but is not widely recognized or utilized in the US. So, it's one more thing you might like to discuss when you SEE YOUR DOC and set off on the path to maintaining normal BP so you can continue to feel great smashing weights for years to come.

CoQ10, Statins, Heart Disease, and

Smashing Weights

Some studies show that coenzyme Q10 (CoQ10) can potentially help with high blood pressure, age-related macular degeneration, and even chronic fatigue syndrome. As an internist who prescribes statins for heart protection, I am also very interested in the cardio-protective effects of CoQ10 when taken with statins.

Statins are a class of prescription drugs designed to lower cholesterol. Some studies have found that up to 25% of patients on statins experience muscle pain and discomfort, a condition known as statin-induced myalgia (SIMS). In addition to muscle pain, people taking statins may sometimes experience nausea, diarrhea, liver and kidney damage, and even increased blood sugar or type 2 diabetes. Statins lower the body's levels of CoQ10. As levels go down, the side effects of statins increase.

In a study published in the *American Journal of Cardiology*, researchers reported that by helping to increase the levels of CoQ10 in the body, CoQ10 supplements seemed to decrease muscle breakdown and reduce pain and discomfort in people taking statins. No dangerous side effects from CoQ10 supplementation have been reported. If you're on a statin and are experiencing side effects, you should discuss with your doctor the potential of adding CoQ10.

The Case of the Heavy Lifter

Recently in my practice, I met with AF, another brother-in- iron. AF came to me after suffering a heart attack. This 44-year- old lifter squats heavier and more often than would seem humanly possible. I spent an interesting two and a half hours with him initially, hearing about his life as a lifter while I examined him and took his health history. After lifting weights for over 20 years, it was only in the past year that AF was diagnosed with a poor lipid panel and hypertension, something we often see in lifters—big men like him. His was yet another case of a heavy-lifting big man who had not been checked regularly by a doctor, and had no idea how important that was, given that his lifting and lifestyle put him at risk for heart disease—that elevated LDL, decreased HDL, hypertension, and being a man (not to mention being a BIG man) added up to enough risks to cause him to develop blocked arteries. One blocked artery is serious enough to earn the dubious distinction of being called the "widow-maker." AF has had to have three drug-eluted stents placed in his heart for life.

Sadly, this case is not all that rare among lifters—lifters who are caught unaware and untreated. I love lifting weights and I love being big. But I love quality of life, too. Is it possible to "win" at both? I believe it is, but only if you take the necessary steps. See an experienced internist who respects and understands your lifestyle and the risks associated with it, and who will *check your lipid panels regularly* to assess whether you are at risk for coronary artery disease. Ask directly about whether you need a cardio-protective dose of statin or proper hypertensive medication.

With the proper care, you can continue to meet your strength goals safely—and feel great while smashing weights for years to come, as I do!!

References

Bookstaver, DA, Burkhalter, NA, Hatzigeorgiou, C. Effect of co-enzyme 10 supplementation on statin induced myalgia, *Am J Cardiol,* 2012 Aug 15;110(4):526-529

23

Gynecomastia

Anabolic-Androgenic steroid (AAS) use is associated with a host of side effects. Some are serious and others are more of a nuisance and can lead to a poor quality of life and cosmetic issues. For example, gynecomastia. Of all the known side-effects of AAS, gynecomastia has to be one of the most infamous among users. On the Internet steroid boards, there are endless numbers of blog posts discussing it; a review of what we actually know about AAS-related gynecomastia should be useful.

Since the early days of AAS use, men have been suffering with anabolic steroid-induced gynecomastia (ASIG)—ironically known as "bitch tits" among men who take these drugs to be big, strong, and to enhance their masculine physiques. Soon after starting these agents, many men develop tender, puffy nipples that resemble a woman's breast. This issue is a common reason why men come to see me.

Let's review the basic physiology of how AAS lead to increased or superphysiologic estrogen levels and resultant gynecomastia. It should be noted that not all AAS that cause gynecomastia do so by

145

direct conversion to estrogen. Some can directly and/or indirectly cause gynecomastia via other specific mechanisms of action (MOA).For example, Anadrol and its relation to inherent estrogenic activity and AAS trenbolone and nandrolone are associated with developing gynecomastia via direct stimulation of breast progesterone receptors, in addition to causing elevated levels of systemic prolactin.

This chapter will focus on the classic AASs that lead to increased systemic estrogen levels and estrogen-based gynecomastia. The normal man has a testosterone/estrogen ratio of about 100/1. Certain types of AAS distort this ratio. The exact MOA of how this happens is unknown, but it is thought that the body tries to maintain balance by increasing systemic estrogen levels in an attempt to counter the elevated testosterone/androgen/susceptible AAS levels and/or that there is some other substrate driven model where a man's body converts testosterone/androgen/susceptible AAS to estrogen in a linear fashion —specific drug/dose and gene dependent, man-per-man. Like many other things in human physiology, this is a multifactorial model. We know that there are many polymorphic genes involved here and that some men can take over 1 gram of testosterone IM per week in addition to other aromatizable AAS and have no signs of gynecomastia, while other men suffer with severe gynecomastia on a low-dose physiologic testosterone regimen. Hence, this topic is controversial not only among physicians and scientists, but also among some of the more cerebral bro-scientists.

What We Know

The human body has an enzyme called aromatase that converts androgens to estrogens and is found in various tissues and cells including adipose, blood vessels, brain, bone, and skin cells. It is thought that when aromatizable steroids like testosterone esters/ suspension, Dianabol, and methyltestosterone interact with aromatase, these AAS agents are converted to systemic estrogen. And as previously stated, the MOA in addition to the degree of conversion has not been fully elucidated. One thing for sure is that men will know when they have reached the threshold for estrogen levels high enough to cause gynecomastia as they start to feel uncomfortable symptoms such as breast and nipple warmth and soreness and tenderness to even the slightest touch of a light shirt. The physical changes that can happen to a man's pec/breast area can cause cosmetic disfigurement and lead to significant embarrassment, making some men feel ashamed about what they have done.

What Can be Done

It goes without saying that the only way to avoid gynecomastia is to not take AAS or even pro-hormones. As with any other drug- related side effects, you need to think deeply before you start taking anabolic steroids. If anything is my take-home message, this is. So many men come to me and say that they wished they would have done more research on AAS prior to starting to use them and that if they did, they either would not have used them or certainly would have used them in a more conservative manner.

As discussed above, there are AAS that are susceptible to aromatization and will convert into systemic estrogen leading to gynecomastia in a drug/dose/man-per-man fashion. The Internet steroids boards talk about two medications that can limit the systemic conversion of androgen/aromatizable AAS to estrogen and block the effects of estrogen at the breast tissue site, respectively: aromatase inhibitors (AIs) and selective estrogen receptor modulators (SERMs). These are medications mainly intended for breast cancer, treating infertility in women and men, and postmenopausal osteoporosis. These medications are very powerful and do work well for what the AAS user is seeking. I am amazed at how the AAS-using community has learned to use these esoteric drugs, presumably without the guidance of a physician. Most experienced AAS users take a two-tier approach to utilizing these drugs: They use AIs mainly for prevention during a AAS cycle, to keep systemic estrogen down; and they use SERMs for "on-

147

the-spot emergency" situations like gynecomastia symptoms. And it seems that these regimens actually can prevent or at least limit the symptoms of gynecomastia. **The problem is that using these medications can also lead to some serious medical issues.**

Yes, the AIs can definitely reduce systemic estrogen levels while one is on testosterone and aromatizable AAS; I have seen that most men who come to me on AAS with AIs—either from the streets or from anti-aging clinics—have estrogen levels at zero! Living with very low or no measurable estrogen is not sustainable, however, and can pose great health risks. Yes, there is less water retention and it is thought that body fat accumulation will be reduced in a physiologic climate of a high androgen/low estrogen state. While this may be true, it is not sustainable, and it certainly isn't safe. The most worrisome things I see regarding the use of AIs are the adverse effects on the cardiovascular system. Anyone who knows me knows my medical mantra: heart protection, heart protection, heart protection. After all, the final rate-limiting step in life will be your heart. AIs are devastating to the good cholesterol, HDL. The fact that many men have a naturally low HDL level is thought to be one of the reasons why men have heart disease earlier than women. I have seen several men on AAS and AIs suffer with blocked arteries.

Apart from the heart issues, I see men complain of sexual issues and depression in addition to erratic behavior while on AIs. We need balanced estrogen in our brains to think correctly and for optimal sex. Another side effect of the use of AIs, although it would be a long-term consequence, is the possibility of medication-induced osteoporosis. I have not seen this in my medical practice, but any man who uses AIs chronically and has low or absent estrogen for years would be at risk for this.

Selective Estrogen Receptor Modulators

The SERMs are a class of drugs that act on estrogen receptors. The specific MOA that makes these agents so unique is that they act as agonists (stimulating activity) in some tissues and antagonists in other tissues (blocking activity). The AAS-using community classically likes to use tamoxifen, which is used medically for breast cancer, for the treatment of osteoporosis and experimentally for the lipids. As stated earlier, this SERM is used to block or deactivate systemic estrogen that is circulating. Remember, AIs block the production of estrogen from the conversion of androgen to estrogen in the body, so when there is sufficient circulating estrogen, breast tissue may be affected and gynecomastia may ensue. There are anecdotal reports that tamoxifen appears to reduce acute symptoms of gynecomastia. However, as with the AIs, I worry about the dangerous side effects and sustainabilty of this drug—especially when used concomitantly with AAS. Because tamoxifen does nothing to reduce systemic estrogen, there is an increase in intravascular fluid (water retention) that can lead to hypertension. Fat storage appears to increase as well with this class of medications. Beyond these side effects is the potential for DVT (blood clots in the lower legs) and PE (blood clots in the lungs that can lead to death) that have been associated with tamoxifen. (Hernandez, 2009) For many years, bro-scientists have promoted tamoxifen as a panacea for preventing the deleterious effects AAS have on lipids—specifically HDL. I can tell you that this notion has never been demonstrated in medical practice, and I would say that using tamoxifen to protect against heart disease while on AAS is nothing less than NUTS!

Clomid is a SERM and works well for men with hypogonadism/TRT—both for men who wish to maintain fertility and for standard TRT. This medication is a classic part of PCT. It has been shown more recently in the literature to be a useful agent to wean men off AAS. (Honen-Yard, 2008) Today, we are seeing more physicians in America using Clomid and other ancillary agents like HCG to help reduce suffering during withdrawal and recovery by men diagnosed with ASIH. In addition to this, there is a place for AIs in the management of men on TRT, as some men who are on appropriate-dose physiologic testosterone replacement can manifest superphysiologic levels of estrogen, despite normal testosterone levels. Remember as discussed above, testosterone/estrogen balance is a multifactorial issue and some men simply have genes for becoming out of balance on TRT. When used in a very cautious and limited fashion, in men who have low heart disease risks—specifically normal HDL levels— the addition of a low-dose AI to TRT can lead to improvements in quality of life via balancing androgen/estrogen levels. When this is done by an expert physician and the qualified patient is observed closely, symptoms of gynecomastia are rare, as are adverse issues related to mood and sexual complaints. It's all about balance and vigilance.

Another very important point regarding TRT and superphysiologic levels of estrogen is the potential for breast cancer. While there is no definitive data indicating that TRT-associated elevations of estrogen lead to breast cancer in men, this is, nonetheless, something that any physician prescribing testosterone has to think about throughout treatment. On a closing note, while I can say that yes, there is a role for these medications in treating the side effects of AAS use, I stress that when they are indicated, it is important that men seek a physician who is knowledgeable about these drugs *as they relate to AAS use*. It is also important to acknowledge the limitations of these drugs. For some men who develop AAS-induced gynecomastia, despite their careful attention to AAS selection and appropriate use of the medications discussed here, it may be necessary to see a plastic surgeon and have excess breast tissue permanently removed.

References

Hernandez, RK et al. Tamoxifen treatment and risk of deep venous thrombosis and... Oct 1;115(19):4442-4449. http://www.ncbi.nlm.nih.gov/pubmed/19569248

Honen-Yard, D. Anabolic steroids: what urologists should know, *Renal and Urology News,* April 2008

24

Cardiovascular Health for All Men

Heart disease is an equal offender of both men and women. However, it is the leading cause of death for men of most racial/ethnic groups in the United States. For Asian American or Pacific Islander men, heart disease is second only to cancer. Between 70% and 89% of sudden cardiac events occur in men. Half of the men who die suddenly of coronary heart disease had no previous symptoms. So, even if you have no symptoms, if you are male, you are still at significant risk for heart disease. The etiology of cardiovascular disease is multifactorial, and the discrete mechanism of action remains elusive and thus beyond the scope of this chapter. The fact I want to drive home here is that, while a number of social factors and life choices also contribute to cardiac disease, primary care medicine can perform an important role in getting men to goal in terms of cardiac health. Because I believe in partnerships between patients and their physicians, I am passionate about the role of education in prevention. So, in addition to reading this chapter, I hope you will review the related video at *www.metabolicdoc.com*.

Make notes as you read and view the information, and take your questions and concerns to your primary care provider. Inform your physician about your lifestyle as well as your symptoms to ensure that the plan you develop to get to goal is a realistic one! There are three main medical risks that lead to cardiovascular disease, and which you and your physician should be monitoring:

- Hypertension and pre-hypertension
- Lipid abnormalities
- Diabetes and impaired fasting glucose (controversial risk, yet very important

Note: NIH guidelines now define hypertension as 130 mmHg and/ or a diastolic blood pressure equal to or greater than 80 mmHg.

If your BP is less than optimal, do something about it, STAT! After smoking cessation and reducing alcohol intake, the first and most obvious issue to address is your body weight. There is a laundry list of evidence relating poor eating habits and being overweight to hypertension and heart disease. The bottom line is that you have to honestly evaluate your behavior and make some changes where needed, which generally means changing your diet and exercise behavior. It's easy to read about diet and exercise, but as a practical matter, it's going to take a sustained effort to get you to goal and keep you there! So I recommend selecting a diet and behavioral changes that you can live with. Yo-yo diets are useless and can not only discourage maintenance but can also be harmful to your health. Developing a realistic and manageable diet and exercise regimen that works for you is more likely to guarantee maintenance and potentially save your life. So, how do you choose from the myriad diet/exercise regimens available? I like a low calorie/carbohydrate Mediterranean diet and I "cheat" with a small meal or two every couple of days. This works for me, and some variation on it may work for your lifestyle. But, remember: one size does NOT fit all.

If, despite having made changes to your diet and exercise habits, you are still in the high pre-hypertensive or hypertensive range, it's time to consider protective supplements and or medications. Here again, there are myriad, potentially confusing, options. For best results, your physician may consult with a qualified naturopathic physician (NP). These professionals are uniquely knowledgeable about dietary and supplemental regimens, including many natural products that have been shown in scientific studies to have positive effects on BP control. Another popular and strongly research-supported approaches is the DASH diet (dietary approaches to stop hypertension), which is essentially a low salt and higher natural potassium diet with a focus on fruits and vegetables. The average man intakes 4,200 mg of salt per day in the US, and the DASH study has shown that reducing salt intake to 2,300 mg and even <1,500 mg per day can substantially reduce BP and save lives. Supplements that have also been reported to reduce BP include omega/fish oil derivations, coenzyme Q10, hawthorn, and high doses of garlic.

For most men with hypertension, and abnormal lipids, a pharmaceutical agent will be required to achieve true and sustained protection. My opinion, and one that is supported by a large body of research, is that physicians should use carefully selected pharmaceutical agents in patient-specific low doses in the early developmental stages of cardiovascular disease—when plaque is building up in a man's arteries. Prescribing blood pressure medications should not be taken lightly, as indicated in the many well-considered medical guidelines such as those listed below regarding the pharmaceutical management of hypertension. In concert with these guidelines, it must always be remembered that addressing hypertension requires a personal approach as well; treating hypertension successfully is as much an art as it is a science. One of the most respected guidelines used world-wide by physicians to aid them in diagnosing and treating hypertension is the *Seventh Report of the Joint National Committee on Prevention, Detection, Evaluation, and Treatment of High Blood Pressure* (JNC 7, 2004).

* Since, in 2017, the Committee made changes to their definition of hypertension, defining this now as 130 mmHg/80 mmHg, some of the following 2004 guidelines may have changed as well. Be sure your physician is up to date.

153

- In persons older than 50 years, systolic BP greater than 140 mmHg is a much more important cardiovascular disease (CVD) risk factor than diastolic BP. * The risk of CVD beginning at 115/75 mmHg doubles with each increment of 20/10 mmHg; individuals who are normotensive at age 55 have a 90% lifetime risk for developing hypertension.

- Individuals with a systolic BP of 120-139 mmHg * or a diastolic blood pressure of 80-89 mmHg* should be considered as pre-hypertensive and require health-promoting lifestyle modifications to prevent CVS.

- Thiazide-type diuretics should be used in drug treatment for most patients with uncomplicated hypertension, either alone or combined with drugs from other classes. Certain high-risk conditions are compelling indications for the initial use of other antihypertensive drug classes (angiotensin converting enzyme inhibitors, angiotensin receptor blockers, beta-blockers, calcium channel blockers).

- Most patients with hypertension will require two or more antihypertensive medications to achieve goal BP (below 140/90 mmHg, or below 130/80 mmHg for patients with diabetes or chronic kidney disease).*

- If BP is >20/10 mmHg above goal BP, consideration should be given to initiating therapy with two agents, one of which usually should be a thiazide-type diuretic.

- In presenting these guidelines, the Committee recognizes that the responsible physician's judgment remains paramount.

There were delays in publishing updates to the 2004 guidelines;

one reason considered plausible by many relates to reported disagreements among the experts about what should be the first-line drugs recommended for the various sub-populations of hypertensive patients. For example, although thiazide diuretics have been the recommended first-line agents thus far, it was thought that this would most likely not be the case in JNC 8. Studies of past evidence-based reviews and of more recent literature on outcomes of thiazide diuretics have caused most hypertension experts to agree that thiazide diuretics should NOT be first-line agents for essential hypertension (a patient who has hypertension without a diagnosis of organic disease; e.g., heart disease, stroke, or diabetes). I agree with this approach and typically do not use thiazide diuretics as first-line for my newly diagnosed hypertensive patients. I will be reviewing the new NIH guidelines regarding this and other protocols I discuss below.

With a quick reminder that this chapter (and, indeed, this book) is intended solely for educational purposes and **not as a substitute for a conversation with your doctor,** I'd like to briefly focus on the two most common medications that I prescribe for my male hypertensive patients. As noted above, I will be reviewing these per new NIH guidelines, as I continually do with all my protocols.

ACE Inhibitors

The first-line drugs I like for most of my hypertensive men who do not have existing heart disease is an ACE-inhibitor (AI). AIs are a group of drugs that cause dilation of blood vessels. They work by reducing BP, and they also have been shown to be effective in protecting the kidneys in patients with diabetes, and hearts in people with existing heart disease. As important, they also provide protection in people without diagnosed heart disease. There is substantial literature supporting blood vessel protection for primary prevention of heart disease and stroke in people without cardiovascular disease, diabetes, or hypertension. That means that these drugs—used only by a physician and personalized for you—can protect your cardiovascular system before you have disease.

Bystolic (Nebivolol Hydrochloride)

Another great medication for hypertension and even high pre-hypertension is a drug called Bystolic (nebivolol hydrochloride). Classified as a third-generation beta-blocker, Bystolic has a novel and unprecedented mechanism of action. Beta-blockers are typically categorized as selective or nonselective to beta receptors. Bystolic may be considered both, depending on the drug's concentration in the body. At low concentrations, typically achieved in extensive metabolizers (the majority of the population) and at doses of 10 mg and below, Bystolic is a beta-1-selective. However, at higher concentrations, in poor metabolizers and at higher doses, Bystolic loses its selectivity and blocks both beta-1 and beta-2 receptors.

Bystolic possesses novel vasoactive factors. It provides vasodilation by releasing endothelial nitric oxide. The vasodilation properties result in an overall positive hemodynamic side-effect profile. I have found that in men with the right medical/personal profile and cardiovascular risks, in addition to a higher resting heart rate—over 80 beats/minute, Bystolic at low doses (2.5-5 mg daily) in addition to an ACE inhibitor works wonders!

I have also discovered that this combination results in well-tolerated and consistent BP control. The usual side effects related to beta-blockers, such as malaise/fatigue, sexual dysfunction, and exercise intolerance are essentially non-existent with low- dose Bystolic, and sexual health can be actually enhanced with this regimen.

References

National Heart, Lung, and Blood Institute. *Seventh report of the Joint*

National Committee on Prevention, Detection, Evaluation, and Treatment of High Blood Pressure (JNC 7), National Heart, Lung, and Blood Institute, NIH Publication No. 04- 5230, August 2004

National Institute of Health. Data from landmark NIH blood pressure study supports important part of new AHA/ACC hypertension guidelines, NIH.gov./news Nov 13, 2017

25

An
Epidemic of
Low-T:
Fact or
Artifact?

As a physician with a general interest in men's health, and a special interest in ASIH, the unique form of hypogonadism that is endemic to AAS use, I have had to inform myself about testosterone and testosterone replacement in every possible aspect. Some of the latest buzz about testosterone is that it ain't what it used to be.

Is it true? Article after article appears now, stating that in a single generation, testosterone levels have fallen significantly in men. Here's are some examples of current thinking:

"Low levels of testosterone impact many aspects of male physiology." states Andre B. Araujo, a research scientist at the New England Research Institutes in Watertown, MA. "This is particularly significant because the ongoing aging of the U.S. male population is likely to cause the number of men suffering from androgen deficiency to increase appreciably." New England

Research Institute scientists a n a l yzed data from almost 1,500 men enrolled in the Boston Area Community Health Survey. The survey tracks people aged 30 to 79 years and compiles data on factors such as testosterone, symptoms of hormone deficiency, and medications that may impact sex hormone levels. Approximately 24% of the men surveyed had low total testosterone and 11% had low levels of free testosterone. Many of the men had no symptoms related to their low testosterone. About 5.6% of the men in this study suffered from symptomatic androgen deficiency. Older men were especially prone: over 18% of men over age 70 met the criteria for this deficiency. Based on these results, the researchers predict that by 2025 there may be as many as 6.5 million American men between 30 and 79 years of age with symptomatic androgen deficiency, an increase of 38% from the year 2000 population estimates. Araujo states, "This study did not assess whether men with symptomatic androgen deficiency are good candidates for testosterone therapy". The Endocrine Society (2012) cautions that "Well-designed, randomized, placebo-controlled trials would be needed to address the risks and benefits of testosterone therapy".

If these experts are correct, it appears that we do have an epidemic of low testosterone (low-T), on our hands. Now the question is what has happened and, more importantly, what can we do about it? Low-T is a medical condition that robs men of their drive for life—including sex, mood, and vitality. This medical state can lead to poor organ health and depression, in addition to a shortened life span. So we better pay attention to what is going on. First, we have to assess the data that has led to this conclusion. It is true that these studies have not been the best in terms of statistical methods, but there is overwhelming clinical and anecdotal data to support their findings indicating that something is wrong; that there is smoke, so there is likely fire.

We have known that men start to lose their "laboratory" testosterone levels of about 1% per year after the age of 30. This does not mean that all middle-aged men are "hypogonadal" or have low-T clinically. The numbers on a lab chart do not represent a man's whole picture. After 15+ years diagnosing and treating men for low-T, I am amazed to see the clinical variation in men in terms of symptoms versus actual lab testosterone levels. What I am saying is that there are plenty of men who present with a low-T lab value; yet, not all of these men complain of the clinical symptoms required to diagnose them as having low-T. On the other hand, I have seen an equally impressive number of men who present with "normal" testosterone lab values who are clinically hypogonadal, despite these levels—hence, the importance of the astute clinician.

Experts are starting to question a strictly lab-defined diagnosis of low-T; clinical features are receiving more attention in the decision about why and who should be treated. As men are becoming more forthcoming about their symptoms, scientists— including me—are recognizing the importance of considering symptoms in our diagnosis and treatment. Men are starting to talk more freely about how they really feel in terms of their sexuality as well as mood and energy; they are expressing directly that they want help, that they expect it. I can also tell you that in my medical practice, in which I have taken care of thousands of men since 2005, men over the age of 75 seldom complain about anything. These are the stoics, hardy men. Many of them have encountered challenges which younger men can only imagine. Many of these men who were born during or before WWII grew up in families that struggled to make ends meet— large families where they had to share; where whining wasn't tolerated. They were accountable. These guys were not designed to "share" their feelings; when they suffer, they do so in a kind of silent dignity, for better or for worse. So, trying to find out how sex is with these guys is like coaxing a tooth out of their heads! When the baby-boomers—and social media —came along, this changed for younger men and even some older ones: there was a lot more talking about such issues. Now the cat comes out of the bag more readily when physicians and researchers screen men for sex-related issues. In my opinion, this new openness is some of what we are now seeing in the current uptick in low-T. It's possible that we are picking up clinical symptoms of low-T that have probably always been there, but which, because of the reticence of men being interviewed in the past, went undetected, particularly if doctors and researchers of that era were also reluctant to press this sensitive issue.

It is also possible to attribute current decreases in testosterone levels to elements of contemporary life. For example, the growing obesity epidemic, exposure to xenoestrogens—plastics, cosmetics, toiletries. (Ever think of what that underarm deodorant is doing to your testosterone level? Did you know that there is actually a very popular type of topical testosterone that men rub on their underarms?) Even in our food supply, we have evidence of estrogens secondary to insecticides and herbicides; high-energy waves from electrical wires, cell phones, and radio wave towers have also been implicated in low-T—what some call today's feminization of men. We can also look at our diets—high in GMO and processed foods that can lead to significant deficiencies in zinc and other minerals, as well as excess stress and elevated cortisol levels and lowered DHEA levels. And, as always, head trauma and chronic medical disease can lead to a low-T state. The most common medical conditions that can lead to low-T are:

- Diabetes and pre-diabetes (insulin resistance)
- Obesity
- Chronic illness
- Depression (can also be the result of low-T)
- Opioid drug use long term
- Alcohol in excess
- Corticosteroid use
- AAS and ASIH

What To Do About Low-T?

Despite all the attention the topic has gotten, it's still difficult to get consensus on who has this condition and how he should be treated—or not. In the clinical practice guidelines provided by various expert medical societies, most now state that there has to be a balance of clinical symptoms related to organic medical disease state(s), in addition to laboratory evaluation. This means that a man has to present to his doctor with classic symptoms associated with low-T, such as malaise/fatigue, poor sexual libido, or erectile dysfunction. Or he has to have a medical condition such as obesity and diabetes or pre-diabetes or other medical condition relating to low-T (see list). All of the expert guidelines agree that the most important clinical features to focus on are symptoms relating to a man's sex drive and sexual performance. All of this data has to be evaluated by an expert physician to decide if a man is a candidate for a trial of physiologic testosterone replacement. The process is a very personal one for each man, who needs to be given adequate time and attention to discuss his symptoms with his doctor, and how these may or may NOT be the result of a low-T state. As I stated above, some men who have lower T lab values, but have "OK" sex lives and are satisfied, will not benefit from testosterone replacement. Reciprocally, there are men with low normal and even at times normal testosterone levels who may benefit from a trial of testosterone replacement. Men who have used AAS in the past are in the group most likely to fall into this latter category. A man should also be counseled on how to improve his overall health. If he can commit to sustained weight loss through diet and exercise, the symptoms that led to low-T can, in many cases, be reversed.

Laboratory Tests to Diagnose Low-T

CBC - complete blood cell count

CMP - comprehensive metabolic panel

LIPID PANEL - total cholesterol, LDL, HDL, and triglycerides

HA1c - hemoglobin A-1C UA - urine analysis

TSH- thyroid-stimulating hormone PSA-prostate specific antigen

Total and free testosterone (LCMSMS; done in the a.m. and can be repeated)

LH and FSH Total estrogen Vitamin D

Starting testosterone replacement as a medical therapy should be taken very seriously. There are risks you should understand before deciding to go this route. Some of these risks have still not been fully elucidated, and their severity remains controversial. I always use evidence-based data to explain each step of my diagnosis and management of the men I work up for low-T. A man should always understand why he is or is not a candidate for testosterone replacement, and what his risks and likely benefits are. A wise man will demand to be seen only by an experienced, board-certified physician who understands and respects the need for such an approach to diagnosing, treating, and managing his condition.

References

Endocrine Society. Declining testosterone levels in men not part of normal aging, *ScienceDaily*, June 23, 2012, www. sciencedaily.com/releases/2012/06/120623144944.ht

26

Hearts and Hormones: Testosterone Replacement and Heart Disease

NEWS FLASH: *The FDA will place an increased warning on all approved prescription testosterone products, requiring manufacturers to notify patients of possible increased risk of heart attacks and strokes in patients taking testosterone, and stating that testosterone therapy is only approved for hypogonadism that has been caused by a specific medical condition and not solely due to age-related low testosterone.*

So, Where Are We Now?

Recent controversy regarding a possible causal link between testosterone and heart disease began in 2013, when *The Journal of the American Medical Association* published an article indicating an association between testosterone therapy and an increase in heart attack, stroke, and death. In the following year, another article reported similar findings. As the media, public interest, and class action suits intensified, Morgentaler and colleagues published their review of the aforementioned studies as well as the extensive literature on testosterone and cardiovascular risks published between 1940 and 2014. These authors found the following:

> *"Only 4 articles were identified that suggested increased [cardiovascular] risks with [testosterone] prescriptions: two retrospective analyses with serious methodological limitations, one placebo-controlled trial with few major adverse cardiac events, and one meta-analysis that included questionable studies and events. In contrast, several dozen studies have reported a beneficial effect of normal [testosterone] levels on [cardiovascular] risks and mortality. Mortality and incident coronary artery disease are inversely associated with serum T concentrations, as is severity of coronary artery disease Testosterone therapy is associated with reduced obesity, fat mass, and waist circumference and also improves glycemic control. Mortality was reduced with [testosterone] therapy in 2 retrospective studies. Several [randomized clinical trials] in men with coronary artery disease or heart failure reported improved function in men who received [testosterone] compared with placebo. The largest meta-analysis to date revealed no increase in [cardiovascular] risks in men who received [testosterone] and reduced [cardiovascular] risk among those with metabolic disease."* (Morgentaler et al, 2015)

The authors concluded, "There is no convincing evidence of increased risks with therapy. On the contrary, there appears to be a strong beneficial relationship between normal testosterone levels and health that has not yet been widely appreciated".

Having taken care of thousands of men on testosterone since 2005, I have clinical evidence that some men are at risk for heart disease if they are not properly treated and monitored. We need to know *which* man is at risk, and *how do we protect him*? And, we need to be clear about who is a candidate for testosterone therapy in the first place.

Whom Do We Treat for Low Testosterone (Low-T)?

In my opinion, a man should only be treated with testosterone if he truly needs it for symptoms, understands the risks, and is willing to work with his physician to monitor his treatment. This means that asymptomatic men, even with low or low normal levels of testosterone, whose goal is "anti-aging" are not candidates. And finally, the decision to treat should be made after open and informed discussion between a man and his physician.

Among the causes of low-T (beyond the normal decrease that accompanies aging) are brain disease, diabetes, damage to a testicle, and—especially in younger men—ASIH. Whatever the underlying cause of low-T, a physician should initiate treatment with the lowest possible dose of testosterone and monitor the patient closely for heart, psychological, and prostate disease. The complex and multifactorial nature of managing men on testosterone requires very specific knowledge about the procedures required to provide TRT safely and effectively. I have seen the immensely improved quality of life that testosterone can bring a man who is managed properly on TRT. I have also seen the tragedy of what can happen to men who have used testosterone unsupervised by a qualified physician.

If you are on testosterone or are considering starting TRT, learn about the potential risks and how these must be medically managed. Interview your physician to determine not only whether he or she is knowledgeable about these, but also whether they will be available to provide the time needed to monitor a safe and effective treatment plan.

References

Morgentaler, A, Miner, MM, Caliber, M, Guay, AT, Khera, M, Traish, AM. Testosterone therapy and cardiovascular risk: advances and controversies, *Mayo Clin Proc,* Feb 2015;90(2):224-251

27

Challenges to Personalizing Testosterone Replacement Therapy With the AAS User

Testosterone replacement therapy (TRT) is one of the recommended protocols for promoting recovery of the hypothalamic- pituitary-gonadal (HPG) axis. It is now known, however, that even with testosterone therapy, hypogonadal symptoms induced by AAS use may persist for many months or more. (2,3,7,8,11) A number of experts recommend treatment with testosterone and other hormonal medications when these steroid-induced hypogonadal symptoms persist. (2,3,7,8,10,11,16,17,18) In some AAS patients, the symptoms are irreversible. (3,17,18) Persistence of hypogonadism even after drug cessation has been explained as "probably the result of long term adaptation to hormones which may involve relatively persistent changes in molecular switches". (1, 10, 15)

Valid and Reliable Signs and Symptoms of HPG Recovery

In 2012, Robert Fitzgerald, Ph.D., Professor of Pathology at the University of California San Diego and AACC representative on the Partnership for Accurate Testing of Hormones, in noting the definitional and measurement dilemmas for diagnosing hypogonadism states, "There are no established reference ranges that people agree on, there's no standardization of the assays, there's really no gold standard for the definition of hypogonadism, and there are no standard sample collection times". (21)

We do not know the thresholds of testosterone level below which clinical features and adverse consequences of androgen deficiency occur. (33) Therefore, diagnosing hypogonadism based solely on lab numbers has increasingly come to be seen as arbitrary. While diagnostic algorithms based on a combination of validated signs and symptoms and population-based lab testosterone reference limits do not yet exist, there is guidance in recent research on hypogonadism which supports the use of clinical symptoms as valid indicators of the disease and of a patient's response to treatment. Equally weighting symptoms and laboratory numbers, Medras and Tworowska stated that continuation of treatment with endocrine medications "is indicated in the presence of persistent clinical symptoms or/and laboratory evidence of HPG dysfunction". (14) Similarly, Morgentaler cautions that "No single [laboratory] number should be used, and symptoms should guide the [hypogonadism] diagnosis. We need to interpret numbers in the context of a man's signs and symptoms". (4) Citing his own cases, Morgentaler provides a warning about the danger of making treatment decisions based solely on "normal" lab numbers, which may not be valid indicators of androgen deficiency in a given individual:

> "Worse (*than the variability among labs*), none of these values were based on symptoms—they were based simply on standard deviation from average levels in the population. In a population with 10% of men with truly low T levels, this approach means you'd miss

three-quarters of them with standard testing. This can have significant impact when a primary care physician, appropriately concerned about the possibility of low T, gets back a "normal" result and falsely concludes that the problem lies elsewhere ."(4)

It is obvious that simply repeating labs would not correct this reliability error in diagnosis. Unlike the lack of consensus on lab numbers to determine adequate testosterone levels, there is strong consensual validation of a group of clinical symptoms as indicators. Zitzmann and Nieschlag (2000) provide examples of symptoms of HPG axis recovery that reflect virtually every discussion in the literature of AAS-induced hypogonadism (ASIH): Restitution of libido, increase in sexual fantasies, and the frequency of erections were considered signs of adequate therapy, while symptoms such as lethargy, inactivity, and depressed mood indicated less than optimum therapy. (18) In these symptoms, clinicians have valid and reliable evidence-based indicators of androgen deficiency in a particular individual.

In 2012, Wartofsky and Handelsman reported that between 20 and 40% of laboratory assays yield errors, typically over- estimating testosterone values. They note that "The 'normal' range has been challenged for several years, particularly at the lower levels, with lack of validity reported for total (as well as free and bioavailable) testosterone. It is believed that it will be another decade before this can be corrected by widespread implementation of standardized state of the art laboratory technology and procedures". (20) Addressing some of these issues recently, Anawalt and colleagues studied 3,672 men and found that while a total testosterone (TT) level greater than 280 ng/dL measured on an accurate, precise assay significantly lowers the likelihood of hypogonadism, a level between 280 and 350 ng/ dL is not sensitive enough to reliably exclude hypogonadism. TT levels must exceed 350 or 400 ng/dL to reliably predict normal free testosterone. (22) In another study based on a community sample of men, Dr. Shalender Bhasin and a group of researchers representing a number of major American and European university centers developed what they described as a "rational basis for categorizing testosterone levels as low or normal." Based

171

on their samples' symptoms, they proposed the following reference ranges: 723.8 ng/dL (mean); 698.7 ng/dL (median/quartile); 348.3 ng/dL (2.5 percentile) .(23) LabCorp, the largest commercial medical lab in the US, has adopted a normal testosterone reference range of 348–1,197 ng/dL. (24)

It is important to recognize that despite the correspondence of these range numbers to eugonadal states in these studies' subjects, study doses and length of treatment do not reflect doses often used—10 to 100 times higher—along with other hormonal products, and over longer periods of time by AAS users. Hence, there is the need for continued caution about extrapolating from these laboratory studies to conditions that might be seen in the field. (29)

Compounding the question of reliability and validity of laboratory levels of testosterone is the variability of actual testosterone levels at peak and trough times during a medication cycle. Currently available testosterone esters initially produce supraphysiological testosterone levels, slowly declining to even pathologically low levels before the next injection. As a result, labs done too early (that is, at "peak" time—early in the adminstration cycle) are likely to reflect supraphysiological levels. (18)   Peak and trough period changes in testosterone levels over the medication cycle are often noticed by patients in terms of marked swings in vigor, sexual activity, and emotional stability. Therefore, the timing of lab samples must also be considered when evaluating numbers. To minimize peaks and troughs while maintaining optimum replacement doses, Zitzmann and Nieschlag recommend that intervals, rather than doses, be adjusted accordingly. (18)

During TRT, 65% of men experience zoospermia, a type of infertility. Avila and colleagues have demonstrated that concurrent use of human chorionic gonadotropin (HCG) preserved fertility, with mean testosterone levels rising from 290 ng/dL before treatment to 960 ng/dL during treatment. HCG adjunct treatment has been found to be necessary for as long as 46 months. (18, 25)

A milestone 5-year study of testosterone thresholds in symptomatic hypogonadal men receiving TRT provided objective evidence to support "the common clinical practice of monitoring the adequacy of androgen replacement therapy by observing how well the presenting symptoms of androgen deficiency are rectified". (33) The authors found that although testosterone level threshold for androgen deficiency is consistent within an individual, it differs "markedly and significantly" between individuals. Genetic polymorphisms, aging, and chronic illness are cited as possible explanations for the differences in threshold testosterone levels. The treatment implication of these findings for hypogonadal AAS users is for recognizing their underlying chronic disease state—ASIH—which may have caused them to develop "normal" testosterone levels that differ from the normal levels of other hypogonadal men.   It is now recognized that men who have become hypogonadal as a result of AAS use represent a subset of hypogonadal men for whom treatment must be adapted with respect to the unique neuroendocrine profile that distinguishes this population. Although studies in which, for ethical reasons, AAS subjects received physiological doses of testosterone over short periods of time have reported findings that can inform treatment of AAS patients, treating men who have used AAS of all kinds, including neuro-toxic substances and in doses 10 to 100 times greater than study samples—cycling these over years, not weeks or months, and presenting with serious AAS related co-morbid medical conditions—will require physicians to be armed with knowledge about the realities of AAS use. By making informed and accurate judgments regarding dependency versus ability to control use (1), and continuing throughout treatment to interpret both signs and symptoms in the context of AAS use (1,2,3,7,8,10,11,15,16,17,18), physicians will be able to provide therapies that not only promptly and adequately address the physiological and psychological sequelae of AAS use, but also to support weaning and cessation (10,13,14).

If, however, the unique symptoms of AAS dependency and its hallmark withdrawal syndrome, hypogonadism, are not recognized and understood by physicians, or if these are disregarded because of reliance on over-generalized ideas about substance abuse, or spurious lab indicators of androgen deficiency, AAS users may be denied relief from painful withdrawal symptoms and timely intervention to restore damaged HPG axis. They may also be denied the opportunity for safely and effectively ending the cycle of use.

In light of the fact that millions of men of all ages, occupations, and social class are now believed to use AAS (5), and that *any* prior AAS use can cause organ damage and induce hypogonadism with its vicious cycle of dependency due to withdrawal syndrome, the number of men potentially harmed is a real and grave concern.

References

1. Brower, KJ. Anabolic androgenic steroid abuse and dependence in clinical practice, *Phys Sports Med,* 2009 Dec;37(4):131-140.

2. Kanayama, G, Brower, KJ, Wood, RI, Hudson, JI, Pope, HG Jr. Issues for DSM-V: clarifying the diagnostic criteria for anabolic androgenic dependence, *Am J Psychiatry,* 2009 Jun; 166(6):642-645

3. Jarow, JP, Lipshultz, LI. Anabolic steroid-induced hypogonadism, *Am J Sports Med,* 1990 Jul-Aug;18(4):429-431

4. Morgentaler, A. Testosterone therapy for life, *Life Extension Magazine,* June 2010

5. National Institute on Drug Abuse (NIDA), *NIH Newsletter*, July 2012

6. Wood, RI. Anabolic androgenic steroid dependency? Insights from animals and humans, *Front Neuroendocrinol,* 2008 Oct;(29) (4):490-506

7. Kashkin, KB, Kleber, HD. Hooked on hormones? An anabolic steroid addiction hypothesis, *JAMA,* 1989 Dec 9;262(22): 3166-3170.

8. Kanayama, KJ et al, Brower, KJ, Wood, RI, Hudson, JI, Pope, HG Jr. Treatment of AAS dependency: emerging evidence and its implications, *Drug Alcohol Depend,* 2010 Jun 1;109(1-3):6-13

9. Caraci, F, Pistarà, V, Corsaro, A, Tomasello, F, Giuffrida, ML, Sortino, MA et al. Neurotoxic properties of the anabolic androgenic steroids nandrolone and methandrostenolone in

primary neuronal cultures, *J Neurosci Res,* 2011 Apr;89(4): 592-600

10.Hochberg, Z et al. Endocrine withdrawal syndromes, *Endocr Rev,* 2003 Aug;24(4):523-538

11.Pope, GH, Brower, KI. Treatment of anabolic-androgenic related disorders, Chapter 17, The American PsychiatricPublishing Textbook of Substance Abuse Treatment, ed. M. Galanter and, H. Kleber, 2008

12.   Spratt, D. Use of performance-enhancing drugs challenges experts, remains a moving target, Endocr Rev, September 2012

13.   Gill, GV. Anabolic steroid induced hypogonadism treated with human chorionic gonadotropin, PostGrad Medicine, 1998 Jan: 74(867):45-46

14. Tayanagi, A et al. Case of androgenic anabolic steroid abuse caused hypogonadotropic hypogonadism, *Hihon Hinyokika Gakkai Zasshi,* 2008 Nov;99(7):729-73

15. Borogowda, K et al. Persistent primary hypogonadism associated with anabolic steroid abuse, *Fertil Steril,* 2001 Jul;96(1):e7-8

16. Zitzmann, M, Nieschlag, E. Hormone substitution in male hypogonadism, *Mol Cell Endocrinol,* 2000 Mar 30;161(1-2):73-88

17. National Institute on Drug Abuse (NIDA). About anabolic steroid abuse, *NIDA Notes,* 2000;15(3)

18. Wartofsky, L, Handelsman, DJ. Standardization of hormonal assays for the 21st century, *J Clin Endocrinol Metab,* 2010 Dec;95(12):5141-5143

19. Collins, G, Fitzgerald, RG. Using total testosterone levels to predict free testosterone, *Clinical Laboratory Strategies,*June 14, 2012. https://www.aacc.org/publications/clinical-laboratory-strategies/2012/using-total-testosterone-levels-to- predict-free-testosterone.aspx

22. Anawalt, B et al. Performance of total testosterone measurement to predict free testosterone for the biochemical evaluation of male hypogonadism, *J Urol,* 2012 Apr;187(4): 1369-1373

23. Bhasin, S et al. Reference ranges for testosterone..., *J Clin Endocrinol Metab*, 2011 Aug;96(8):2430-2439

24. Pencina, M, Jasuja, GK, Travison, TG, Coviello, A, Orwoll, E, LabCorps. Q & Testosterone reference intervals, www.LabCorps.com/ assets 11476, 2017. Reference ranges for testosterone in men generated using liquid chromatography tandem mass spectrometry in a community-based sample of healthy nonobese young men in the Framingham Heart Study and applied to three geographically distinct cohorts. *J Clin Endocrinol Metab,* 2011 Aug; 96(8):2430-2439

25. Avila, D, Gittens, PR, Hwang, K, Weedin, JW, Rumohr, JA, Lipshultz, LI. Low dose human chorionic gonadotropin prevents azoospermia and maintains fertility in hypogonadal men on testosterone replacement therapy, *Fertil Steril,* 2010;94(Suppl 4):128-121

26. Kuhn, CM. Anabolic steroids, *Recent Prog Horm Res,* 2002;57:411-434

27. Kanayama, G et al. Illicit anabolic-androgenic steroid use, *Horm Behav,* 2010 Jun:58(1):111-121

28. Kanayama, G, Brower, KJ, Wood, RI, Hudson, JI, Pope, HG Jr.

Anabolic androgenic steroid dependency: an emerging disorder, *Addiction,* 2009 Dec;104(12):1966-1978

29. Menon, DK. Successful treatment of AAS-induced zoosperm, *Fertil Steril,* 2003 June;79(Suppl 31):141-143

30. Tan, RS et al. An unusual case of vascular hypogonadism treated with clomiphene citrate and testosterone replacement, *Andrologia,* 2009 Feb;41(1):63-65

31. Kelleher, S et al. Blood testosterone threshold for androgen deficiency symptoms, *J Clin Endocrinol Metab,* 2004 Aug; 89(8):3813-3817

28

Big Mike

In this chapter, I will present the anonymized case of a patient who represents a special kind of American hero to me—a strength athlete and medical hero. Many of us live the mantra of cardiac protection and can stack the deck in our favor by following the rules, but none of us—no matter how jacked—are immune to cancer. Not even Big Mike, as I will fictitiously call him.

Big Mike, age 43, is a good natured red, white, and blue American stud from the Midwest. Mike matured from a "quiet and chubby" kid into a confident young man once he found his place in the world of sport. He did a few seasons of other sports in high school, but when he found powerlifting there was no stopping him, and before long he had developed himself into a hard- nosed lifter. After high school, his dream was to eventually have his own construction company and to relocate to a place where more work—and sunshine—was available than in the Midwest.

The focus and strength he had developed as a dedicated lifter made the work easy for Mike, whose sport had also taught him the importance of observing safety precautions. This approach made him popular with his coworkers and respected by his bosses. With his career and life as a lifter well underway, Mike married his high school sweetheart and moved to the South where he had an opportunity to start his own company. Bliss.

Here, however, is where the fairy tale falters. Things start to fade when Mike, a paragon of good health who never had more than a cold in all his adult life, presented himself to his doctor with what he thinks is a chronic sinus infection. It's already cost him days off the job. The doctor finds huge swollen lymph nodes on both sides of Mike's neck. His doctor conducted several tests and then, being concerned, referred Mike to a specialist. In spring of 2011, Mike's ENT doctors did an excisional biopsy of the abnormally large lymph nodes. Their diagnosis was non-Hodgkin's lymphoma. Mike remembers everything that was whirling around in his head when he heard this. Was it from Lyme? He remembered the tick bite he'd had last summer at the beach. Is it my job? Were there any dangerous chemicals at the worksites? My food? Couldn't be—I eat only the best—organic, too. What does this mean? Am I going to die? I feel fine.

During a his visit to an oncologist, Mike was told, "You're what is considered Stage 4, but it's a treatable—though not curable cancer. We recommend chemotherapy, right away. If you don't do the chemotherapy, you have maybe a year to live."

In one week, Mike had an appointment in the Northeast at one of the best cancer centers in the world. The oncologist concurred with the diagnosis of NHL Stage 4 (bulky follicular B-cell type), but felt that the chemo could be put off for a while and that Mike would be a candidate for a "watchful waiting process." He ordered Mike to immediately stop using any AAS or supplements he had been using in his weightlifting regimen. Mike complied and immediately began to make his plan. He was ready to battle this disease, and he knew that chemo was going to be part of that battle plan. But, knowing what chemo could do to the body, he was determined to stack the deck against side effects and not let them further destroy the body he had worked all his life to build (you brothers-in-iron can certainly relate to that). Mike researched all potential alternative/holistic treatments to see what could fortify him for the fight of his life. If you want to know anything about alternative therapies for non-Hodgkin's lymphoma, just call Mike. He's a walking naturopathic encyclopedia. His research into alternative therapies convinced him to go on intravenous vitamin C three times a week and to add in lymph massages, infrared sauna therapy, and colonics to fortify himself for what was ahead.

He continued to work and train as usual. At first he felt great in the gym, as he was smashing over 400 pounds on the incline bench, but eventually it got harder and harder to train. A long- time reader of my Anabolic Doc column, Mike decided to make the journey to Connecticut to see me. I remember thinking, "This man has a bad form of lymphoma and he's coming to me for help? He has some of the world's foremost cancer experts to guide him. What's going on here?" When Mike explained his reasons for coming to see me, his words echoed those I have heard from many men: He came to me because, he said, none of his physicians understood that at his core he was a bodybuilder, and that this was crucial for the healer to not only understand, but to support while he was healing. It was clear that it was from this core that Mike drew on the spiritual power to wage war with cancer cells. He came to me as a man, a lifter, and a patient looking for support. He was prepared to do the heavy lifting for his treatment himself. I wondered what role, in addition to his cancer, his sudden withdrawal from AAS and supplements had also played in the symptoms he was reporting. I conducted my History and Physical exam and after my laboratory review, I discovered that Mike was severely hypogonadal. It was likely that sudden AAS withdrawal as well as the stress of his disease, had caused Mike's testosterone levels to plummet.

Mike agreed to let me call his oncologist to discuss the possibility of testosterone replacement therapy. I made the call that afternoon and found his doctor very professional and, of course, brilliant in terms of cancer treatment, as I knew he would be. What was amazing to me was that he had no input—either good or bad—on instituting TRT in a patient with non-Hodgkin's lymphoma. I find it interesting that one of the best cancer docs on Earth had no position on cancer treatment of this kind while on replacement testosterone, given that testosterone is one of the best medicines for gaining strength and building up bodies, not to mention that so many men—potentially including patients with Mike's diagnosis—are already on these regimens.

We started Mike on testosterone replacement therapy and soon he reported feeling good again—good enough to sustain his alternative treatment regimen and his strength training, as well as having a good quality of life in many other areas. A year later, it was time to start chemo. His lymph nodes were increasing in size, as were his liver and spleen. His liver enzymes had skyrocketed. He was started on a 6-month chemo regimen that would test any man, rock-solid guys like Mike included. As the months rolled on, Mike would call me and say, "This chemo is no joke, but I'm feeling OK, Doc." And throughout this period, he lived like few other patients on chemotherapy live: he worked 3 weeks out of every month and continued to train hard. After each treatment, he would go home and "go to war with the weights," challenging himself to make sure he was still strong. After multiple cycles of chemo, Mike came out on top. His current scans show no active cancer.

After all Mike has been through, when he reflects on his journey, he says he would like everybody who has to fight cancer to understand a few basic truths about what got him through it. First, he says, was the importance of preserving his source of physical, mental, and spiritual strength—maintaining his bodybuilding routine—coupled with support from family, friends, and his medical team for the plan he'd made for himself. Mike acknowledges that, as much of a poison as chemotherapy is, it does the job of killing the cancer cells. That's the good part of the chemo. But its undeniable assault on the rest of the body needs to be addressed, as well. This is where mainstream medicine has something to learn from alternative medicine—and from patients like Mike, the real experts on their own lives and what makes life worth living, worth fighting for. No one will argue that Mike's successful outcome is anything less than a miracle of modern allopathic medicine, but we have to also consider the contribution of his pre-treatment with alternative therapies, and that of TRT to his ability to maintain a satisfying quality of life throughout his illness. Mike's case demonstrates how having medical support to maintain adequate testosterone levels during the stress of serious illness can contribute to a good treatment outcome by supporting a man's physical and mental health, and providing a quality of life satisfying enough to sustain him throughout his ordeal.

Now Mike is back at work. He won a lucrative contract to come up to New York City to work on rebuilding those gorgeous Freedom Towers in lower Manhattan. God bless you, Mike, for what you do, and for what you have taught us, bro!

29

The Bigger, Younger
Steroids Problem

Dear Editor:

Each year, drug testing and whistle blowing provides more evidence of systematic, state-sponsored Russian doping. Headlines about this and about US Olympians and professional athletes who also cheat transfix readers. It's the perfect opportunity to tell the bigger story of anabolic steroid (AAS) use—the story closer to home, the one that affects millions, including school age children. And yet, this Everyman part of the doping story has yet to capture the media's attention. Their narrow focus on star athletes may simply reflect media-as-business, with primary concern for the financial bottom line; it is nonetheless disappointing when any influential institution overlooks an opportunity to perform an important public service.

As the steroids epidemic involving ordinary Americans grows, I continue to be puzzled about why the media has overlooked this aspect. Isn't the spectre of 4 million ordinary Americans playing Russian roulette with their health indicative of a burgeoning public health crisis? How is it that our institutions, including the media, don't seem to be seeing this gathering storm?

Perhaps a retrospective look at the current opioids/heroin crisis would be instructive: Full recognition of a brewing opioid/heroin epidemic did not come until several years after there were already developments which foreshadowed it. For example, between 2005 and 2009, heroin imports from Mexico and Colombia had increased six-fold, to nearly 50 metric tons; and by 2011, prescriptions for opioids had already nearly tripled (Frontline, 2014). Yet it was several years before the problem signaled by these red flags prompted intense multi-media and government attention.

Is there a specific critical mass that has to accrue before our institutions begin to mobilize, to bring their full resources to bear on a public health issue? High death toll? Extreme financial costs? When the tipping point is reached, we mount full court intervention to contain the epidemic, and in our "crisis autopsies", identify harbingers that should have been recognized much earlier, along with the systems that failed to recognize or respond to these. Changes are made, and there are sincere calls from every sector for a pre-emptive strike —"next time".

The problem is that "next times" seldom look like their predecessors.

In this book, I have tried to describe what makes this "next time" unique; to bring attention to a number of indicators of an AAS epidemic hiding in plain sight, the dangers attending it, and some gaps in systems that might otherwise limit harm. I have also attempted to make the case that current efforts to address this brewing epidemic have not only failed, but may actually have been counterproductive: The prevailing emphasis on AAS use as virtually exclusively a law enforcement and moral issue has driven use farther underground, distancing users even from physicians whose help they require. The fact that the steroids industry is booming (Epstein, 2015) is testimony to this failed strategy. The incredible ease with which AAS can be procured through the Internet has been an undeniable accelerant to increasing use of both illicit steroids and legal over-the-counter supplements that actually contain steroids and untold other harmful substances. While this epidemic has reached across all sectors of American society, the involvement of school age children should be reason enough to take a closer look at what's going on here.

In addition to the number of private and government studies which have documented the involvement of school age children in AAS use., one has only to look at the many online AAS forums to see evidence of young people seeking information and advice about using and about moving on to even more potent drugs and protocols. (McBride et al, 2016).

Yet, in 2015, the National Institute on Drug Abuse reported that "fewer school-age kids are using steroids now". My reading of the data from a variety of other reliable sources does not elicit so comforting a conclusion, however.

While they vary somewhat across studies, the numbers and the facts surrounding student use continue to be alarming. For example, in 2015, the FDA stated that the frequency of steroid use in teenagers is "far greater than many would guess", and the Mayo Clinic reported that as many as 1 in 20 teenagers use steroids to increase muscle mass. According to the Monitoring the Future Study (2016), steroids are used by 1.0% of 8th graders, 1.2% of 10th graders, and 2.3% of 12th graders. In 2013, the FDA estimated that among these high school users, each year 375,000 young men and 175,000 young women are using steroids at the level of abuse.

These school age users' motivations for using AAS are especially troubling. In their 2017 website fact sheet, the Taylor Hooton Foundation reported that among the 1.5 million students, with a median age of 15, who report using steroids, many continue to believe that these drugs are not dangerous. These studies also found that 57% of the students they interviewed said that they would still take these drugs to meet their goals, even if doing so would shorten their life. An astounding 65% of student users described their reasons for using as "improving their looks."

If all that these young people have to guide them are lectures stressing the illicit nature of AAS and sensational reports of high-profile professional sports doping, the likely take home message for them is that doping works, or elite athletes wouldn't do it; and as long as you have no medals to lose, why not try it. It can make you look really good.

References

Brower, KJ. Anabolic androgenic steroid abuse and dependence in clinical practice, *Phys Sportsmed,* 2009 Dec;37(4): 131-140

Cohen, J. A league of their own: demographics, motivations and patterns of use of 1,955 male adult non-medical anabolic steroid users in the United States, *J Int Soc Sports Nutr,* 2007 Oct 11;4:12

Engel, R, Petropoulos, A. Whistle blowers fear for their lives after cyber attack, NBC News, Aug. 28, 2016

Epstein, D. Everyone's Juicing, *ProPublica,* Sep. 17, 2015

U.S. Food and Drug Administration. Teens and steroids: a dangerous combo, *FDA Consumer Updates,* 2013

Frontline. The drug wars, *WGBH Educational Foundation,* 2000

Hochberg, Z, Pacak, K, Chrousos, GP. Endocrine withdrawal syndromes, *Endocr Rev,* 2003 Aug;24(4):523-538

Honen-Yard, D. Anabolic steroids: what urologists should know, *Renal and Urology News,* April 10, 2008

Medscape.com. Steroids use among non-athletes. Why?, *Medscape,* Aug 22, 2016. http://Medscape.com/viewarticle/867629

National Institute on Drug Abuse. Monitoring the future, 2015 Survey Results, December 2015

McBride, JA et al. The availability and acquisition of illicit anabolic androgenic steroids and testosterone preparations on the Internet, *Am J of Men's Health*, May 11, 2016. pii:1557988316648704

Pope, G, Brower, KJ. Treatment of anabolic-androgenic steroid related disorders, Chapter 17, in *The American Psychiatric Publishing textbook of substance abuse treatment*, eds. M. Galanter, H. Kleber, 2008

Rahnema, C, Lipshultz, LI, Crosnoe, LE, Kovac, JR, Kim, ED. Anabolic steroid induced hypogonadism: diagnosis and treatment, *Fertil Steril*, 2014 May;101(5):1271-1279

Talih, F, Fattal, O, Malone, D Jr. Anabolic steroid abuse: psychiatric and physical cost, *Cleve Clin J Med*, 2007 May;74(5):341- 344, 346, 349-352

Taylor Hooton Foundation. Taylor Hooton Foundation Expands National Reach, Fact Sheet, August 2017